*Survivor S~~~~
f(*

1st Edition

Shalin Shah
Author, Medical Student

Kristyn Czapkowski
Illustrator

Michael L. Tizol
Graphic Designer

Disclaimer

The information provided in this book is presented solely for educational purposes. While honest efforts have been used in preparing this book, the author and publisher make no representations or warranties of any kind and hereby disclaim any liabilities of any kind, to all parties, with respect to the accuracy or completeness of the contents. The author and publisher do not assume any liability to any party for any loss, damage, or disruption caused by errors or omissions, whether such errors or omissions result from negligence, accident, or any other cause. The information in this book is meant to supplement, not replace, proper orthopedics education.

To all my family, friends, and mentors who have supported me during my endeavors

Table of Contents

Preface

As a 3rd year medical student, I realized that I had decided fairly late in my academic career (compared to many of my colleagues) regarding my interest in orthopedic surgery. In my understanding, many students go to medical school with the sole desire to practice orthopedics, meaning they have some sort of familiarity with the discipline that the average student does not. Appreciating the competitiveness of the field, I knew it was compulsory to flourish on my elective rotations. I essentially put all of my energy toward this desire to learn orthopedics and contacted current resident physicians, attended didactics and fracture conferences, joined research projects, went to national meetings, and took notes on everything I possibly could. I was recommended a few of the standard books used by students, but I realized that there was no source particularly targeted at introducing the field to medical students. Rather, students have been extracting information from resident level books and over time figuring out a starting point for their learning. Considering that orthopedics is a subject that is not comprehensively taught during medical school, I thought it would be in the best interest of medical students to create a source that introduces some of the basic terminology and clinical principles. This will allow a student to develop a solid foundation upon which to build his or her orthopedic knowledge.

History/ Notes/ X-ray Basics

A historical perspective of orthopedics may help you better grasp an understanding of where the field comes from and how it is evolving. The term "orthopaedics" is derived from two Greek words, *orthos*, meaning "straight," and *paidios* meaning "child." This term was originally intended to describe the methods for managing deformities in children. Through time the Greeks, Romans, and Renaissance physicians began to take increasing interest in such deformities as these children were oftentimes ostracized from society. It was since those ancient times that there was recognition of the importance of correcting proper bone length and alignment. Over the following years various discoveries and innovations in the medical field have evolved, with one of the most noteworthy being the total hip replacement in the 1960's by Dr. John Charnley from England. (If you watch a hip replacement, you will notice that there is an important tool used in the approach termed a "charnley retractor").

As you know, the field of orthopedics relies greatly on radiographs and imaging to guide both diagnosis and management. To touch on its history, German physicist Wilhelm Roentgen is recognized as the father of the x-ray. He discovered this in 1895 when he stumbled upon and began studying fluorescent electrical discharges around some tubes in his lab. He took the first recognized x-ray about a week after his discovery, which was of his wife's hand, displaying her bony anatomy as well as her wedding ring. Within months of his discovery, surgeons began utilizing radiographs to guide their work. About a year later in 1896, Thomas Edison developed the fluoroscope, which is now a standard in medical x-ray examinations, particularly in the operating room.

Pre-op/ post-op notes – As a medical student, it is compulsory to become proficient with appropriate documentation. As taking a history and performing a physical exam come with practice, you will learn the importance of documentation in the medical world. Although legal issues are enough of a reason to learn it well, communicating findings with other healthcare providers is just as consequential.

There are several factors to take into consideration when assessing an orthopedic patient, whether it be preoperatively or postoperatively.

Here's a start: Looking at the area of focus, assess the integrity of the skin and soft tissue. Be sure to describe any lacerations, ecchymosis, swelling, or deformities. It is also a good habit to assess the compartments, as the development of compartment syndrome is an orthopedic emergency (described later). The appearance of the wound/incision should be noted for any erythema or purulence, and described whether it is intact or not. A sensory and motor exam should *always* be done for the potential affected nerves, along with assessing the local pulses and ranges of motion (See index for examples of nervous supply). Muscle strength of specific muscle groups should be documented. [This means you must know the grading of muscle strength on the scale of 0-5. This also means that you must know your anatomy very well!]. If there are any orthopedic devices being used, they should also be described by the type and status, along with patient tolerance. For example, if any splint, cast, brace or traction is being used, it should be noted. Post-operative notes should always include how many days after the procedure the patient is being assessed, as there are different expectations regarding progression, as well as complications (i.e. John Doe is a 45-year-old male, status post total knee arthroplasty, post-op day (POD) #2). Patients that have lower extremity procedures are especially prone to developing DVTs, with hospitalization and immobilization being additional risk factors. For this reason, we place most of our patients on anticoagulants. Make sure you note which form of anticoagulation or other DVT prophylaxis is being used for the patient! Therefore it is also essential to note any lab results corresponding to the anticoagulation medication being given (ex: INR for those on Coumadin). Patients are oftentimes being cared for by several different services, so coordinating care is crucial in the proper management of our patients. As improvement of functional status is the objective for orthopedic surgeons, physical

Muscle Strength Scale
0/5 – no movement
1/5 – twitching
2/5 – movement with gravity ELIMINATED
3/5 – movement against gravity
4/5 – movement against gravity with resistance (less than normal)
5/5 – normal strength

therapy/occupational therapy should be mentioned in the note. Also related to this, and considering that some procedures may be of greater caliber, pain control is important to manage. If a patient is in pain, how are they going to progress in their therapy? A mnemonic to help remember what to include in the "Plan" part of the SOAP note are the 5 P's [Pain control, PT/OT, PE (DVT prophylaxis), discharge Planning, Pus (antibiotics)].

Everybody has his or her own way of documenting a SOAP note. Below is an example of a progress note on an orthopedic patient:

S: Patient seen at bedside, has no current complaints. Patient states pain is well-controlled, described as 4/10. Patient denies any nausea, vomiting, chest pain, SOB. Patient denies having any bowel movements since surgery, but states his appetite is fine. Patient denies any overnight events.

O: *Vital signs*
   Pertinent Laboratory/Radiographic findings
   Physical therapy progress from the day

   Physical Exam: <u>Right Lower Extremity</u>
           Incision is clean/dry/intact
           Compartments are soft to palpation
           Sensations grossly intact L2-S1
           Strength 5/5 in Tibialis anterior, flexor hallucis longus,
                   extensor hallucis longus, and gastrocnemius/soleus
           Pulses +2 at dorsalis pedis and posterior tibial arteries

A/P: 45-year-old male, POD # 2 of Right total knee arthroplasty
           1.   Pain control – IV Dilaudid
           2.   PT/OT – Weight-bearing as tolerated
           3.   DVT prophylaxis – Low-molecular weight heparin
           4.   D/C Planning – to subacute rehabilitation tomorrow

X-ray basics – Through experience and practice, it is important to acquire the skills of both interpreting and presenting radiographs. Like all things, a systematic approach should be used to ensure you are not missing anything. Firstly, it is important to confirm the name, date, and age of the patient. Then you should orient yourself to what you are looking at. For example, consider the view, consider what part of the body are you looking at (is it the right or left side), and does it represent a skeletally mature or immature individual. The projection/view, for example, can be anterior-posterior (AP) projection, lateral view, oblique view etc. You should always use at least 2 views to sufficiently interpret a radiograph (**1 view = no views**). Also remember to be mindful of the joints above and below the affected area, particularly in trauma patients as they may also be affected. *Make sure you have assessed whether the area of injury is neurovascularly intact and keep in mind the mechanism of injury.* After this, take a moment to assess the radiograph for any abnormalities or significant variances of the bony anatomy, joints, and soft tissue structures if visible. Consider taking bilateral films as it may point out normal versus abnormal anatomical variants. Also, always order a radiograph post-reduction of a fracture/dislocation.

The location of the lesion is always important to note. Long bones are normally broken down into regions termed the epiphysis, diaphysis, metaphysis, and physis. The epiphysis is the end of the bone (forming the joint), the diaphysis is the shaft of the bone, and the metaphysis is in between those two. In children the physis (growth plate) is an essential determinant in fracture type and management, as described later.

It is important to include the particular demonstrating features:
- Number and type of views
- Skeletal maturity
- Type of Fracture (transverse, comminuted, spiral, butterfly fragment, torus/buckle, oblique, segmental etc.)
- Intra- or Extra-articular
- Displacement
- Angulations
- Shortening/Overlap/ "Bayonetting"
- Rotation
- Soft tissue swelling

For example, an x-ray may be read as follows: "There are 2 views, AP and lateral, of a right hip, in a skeletally mature individual, demonstrating a subcapital femoral neck fracture, that is partially displaced."

Or another example: "This is an AP view of a right ankle in a skeletally mature individual, demonstrating a minimally displaced oblique fracture of the distal fibula. There is no medial clear space widening. The syndesmosis appears to be intact. "

Although classification systems are utilized for most fracture patterns, do NOT go into this when originally presenting an x-ray. Simply describe what you see in a concise manner.

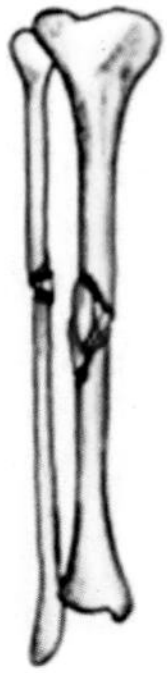

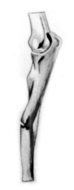

Figure 1: Comminuted fx of tibial shaft and fibula

Note: You will very often hear the terms **"varus"** and **"valgus"** in describing fractures, and it is important you add them to your medical jargon. Simply, varus means the apex of the deformity is away from the midline, whereas valgus means the apex of the deformity is with the apex toward the midline. You will pick this up with practice.

Fractures are described by their resulting damage, using terms such as **comminuted, transverse, oblique, spiral,** and **simple**. A simple fracture means that the bone is broken in two pieces, whereas a comminuted fracture

Figure 2: Greenstick fx

is broken into several pieces (as what happens when a glass plate is dropped on marble and shatters). A comminuted fracture represents high-energy trauma, and subsequent greater soft tissue damage, warranting further investigation of the local musculoskeletal structures.

An example of a greenstick fracture is seen in Figure 2, which is seen in children where the bone bends rather than completely breaks. Fracture **angulation** is important to understand, and describes the way the bone is broken. It is named by the direction of the distal fragment of the break, or by the apex of the angulation. For example, a fracture may be described as having "dorsal angulation" or the same fracture described as "apex volar" (see Figure 3).

It is also important to keep in mind that emergency department consults will make up a significant part of your training. It is in your best interest to handle these cases as efficiently as possible. Generally when returning a page, one should ask 3 simple questions relating to the orthopedic injury that can help stratify its urgency:

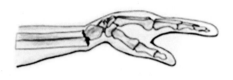

Figure 3: Dorsal angulation, apex volar ("Colles' fracture")

1. Is it open or closed?
2. Is the patient neurovascularly intact?
3. Are there any additional views/radiographs needed?

General Principles

With over 200 bones in the body and the responsibility of managing the elaborate musculoskeletal system, the field of orthopedics is presented with a broad spectrum of disorders. Fractures are a significant aspect of the practice, and so for the importance of patient management and communication, various terms and classification systems are used. You will learn that fractures are grouped by their anatomic location and classified based on severity and specific characteristics.

A quality classification system should have the following features:
- Describes the injury
- Directs treatment
- Describes the prognosis
- May be useful for research
- Has satisfactory inter-observer and intra-observer reliability

In brief, there are different types of bone that make up the human skeleton. Bone may be composed of compact (cortical) bone, which is strong, dense, and makes up 80% of the skeleton. This includes the diaphyses of long bones. Cancellous bone on the other hand is weaker and more flexible, but has a greater blood supply. _Cancellous_ bone is more severely affected than cortical bone in patients suffering from osteoporosis.

As mentioned earlier, one of the primary factors to consider is whether the fracture is open or closed. An **open fracture** is one in which the skin is broken, exposing the fracture to contamination. Thus, they generally require urgent treatment with IV antibiotics (1st generation **cephalosporin**, adding **aminoglycosides** depending on extent, with further contamination adding **Penicillin**) and possible surgical debridement. On exam, a clue to the fracture being exposed to the outside environment is if you notice _fat droplets in the blood_ (from bone marrow fat). When called down to the Emergency Department for an open fracture, the first things to ask about are the status of tetanus and antibiotics.

The administration of tetanus prophylaxis is essential for such exposed fractures. If it is a polytrauma situation (as many open fractures are), there are specific radiographs that you must ask for; these include a lateral C-spine, a chest x-ray, and a pelvic x-ray. If operative irrigation and debridement is necessary, then the patient should be prepared as NPO (nothing by mouth), appropriate blood work (i.e. CBC), consent, ECG, and chest x-ray.

Open fractures can be classified according to the **Gustilo & Anderson classification**, which goes as follows:
- **Type I** – Wound is **< 1cm** in size with minimal bone and soft tissue comminution
- **Type II** – Wound is **1-10 cm** in size with moderate soft tissue injury and moderate comminution
- **Type III** (broken down into 3A, 3B, and 3C; all of which have severe soft tissue damage and comminution)
  - **A** – Adequate amount of soft tissue coverage of the bone
  - **B** – Inadequate soft tissue coverage
  - **C** – Associated vascular injury

This classification involves the patient being evaluated *intraoperatively*. This means that a patient may come in with a Grade 2 injury, but once you take them to the OR and debride them appropriately, the wound will increase in size and become a Grade 3, and therefore the wound is classified as a Gustilo & Anderson Grade 3.

Closed fractures, on the other hand, are not exposed to the environment, and tend to heal quite well. Regardless of fracture type, muscle viability is important to take into consideration. This is of particular importance when one is considering a compartment syndrome and there is risk of tissue necrosis. Muscle viability can be assessed using the 4 C's (**C**olor, **C**onsistency, **C**apacity to bleed, and **C**ontractility) as when a fasciotomy is performed. Normal muscle is characterized as beefy red in color, firm, and responsive to a forceps pinch (contractility). Contractility is the most sensitive sign, and this can be done by using low-voltage electro cautery or by slowly tapping the tendon.

Another classification system that affects management in the field of traumatology is the **Tscherne classification of closed fractures.** This is broken down as follows:

0   No appreciable soft tissue injury
1   Superficial abrasions or contusions
2   Significant muscle contusion – *high risk for compartment syndrome*
3   Extensive crushing of soft tissues. Vascular disruption or compartment syndrome may be present

One of the most important considerations with open and even closed fractures is the associated soft tissue envelope. The loss of this envelope may further affect fracture immobilization. As a surgeon had once told me, "a fracture is a soft tissue injury associated with a break in the bone." He was simply depicting that soft tissue is of utmost importance in fractures as it has the ability to mandate healing potential from the extra-osseus/periosteal blood supply.

When there is disruption of the anatomy around a bone or joint, certain deforming forces will cause the anatomy to be altered in its normal alignment. This will generally need to be fixed, and the appropriate term is "reduced." **Reduction**, which is the process of positioning the fracture or dislocation back to its normal alignment, can also be described as "closed" or "open." This simply refers to the use of operative manipulation via making an incision. For example, using a splint or even percutaneous pinning would be considered closed reduction, compared to opening the skin to fixate the bone with a plate and screws. When fractures are displaced from their normal anatomic position, it is important to reduce them for the following reasons: **1).** Reduction *decreases the risk of neurovascular damage.* **2).** *Minimizes soft tissue injury* **3).** *Decreases pain/discomfort* (Additional analgesia and muscle relaxation is usually needed during the process). **4).** Facilitates transportation of the patient. **5).** Brings the limb out to its correct length thereby preventing muscle shortening and contraction. When considering reduction, attempts should be made to restore the bone's *length, rotation,* and *angulation.* Remember to order post-reduction radiographs after operative or non-operative treatment to ensure that your goals were reached, and <u>always</u> reassess neurovascular status.

Three important measures to keep in mind when reducing a dislocation or a fracture in the Emergency department are as follows:

1. Accentuate the deformity
2. Place Traction
3. Reverse the mechanism of dislocation

So for example, a distal radius fracture with dorsal angulation, apex volar can be reduced by placing traction on the distal fragment, along with a volar force to that fragment. You will understand this better once you read the rest of the chapter.

When non-operative management would be inadequate, it is important to keep in mind the goals for surgical treatment. These are based on the international AO principles and include:

1). Anatomic reduction of all fragments

2). Securing fracture fixation

3). Preserving the blood supply and respecting the integrity of the surrounding soft tissue and

4). Early range of motion

Generally speaking, open reduction is indicated when there is an open fracture, failed closed reduction, neurovascular compromise, or intra-articular fracture. Although it may be necessary, there are potential complications. These include infection, mal/nonunion, blood loss, and even the possibility of creating a new fracture.

Joint involvement is also important in determining prognosis and management of orthopedic injuries. A fracture involving the articular surface poses an increased risk for future development of

15

osteoarthritis. Therefore, precise reduction is important and often requires operative management to obtain functional results.

If a patient ensues a traumatic fracture, the reason it is important to get imaging of the joints below and above is not only to assess for additional fractures, but to also consider any prostheses that may be in place. Periprosthetic fractures are also an entity that must be considered, and the treatment depends on several factors including the location, stability, bone stock, and the medical condition of the patient. These fractures can be organized using the **Vancouver classification:**

> **Type A:** Fracture in peri-trochanteric region
> **Type B:** Fracture around or just distal to stem
> > **B1:** Stable stem
> > **B2:** Loose stem, adequate bone stock
> > **B3:** Loose stem, inadequate bone stock
> **Type C:** Fracture well below the stem

Bone healing can occur in two ways, as does skin healing. There are "primary" and "secondary" mechanisms. Primary bone healing is when the surgeon causes intimate contact of the cortices of the bone. This generally requires internal fixation as there should not be any soft tissue in between fragments. This is also termed "rigid fixation" since bone heals directly to bone. Secondary bone healing is when there is *callus formation* by the body to bridge the fracture. Callus formation is the process of a fibrous matrix being laid down that eventually transitions to cartilage and then to bone. Generally speaking, this is what happens during casting of a fracture.

Several patient factors can affect the prognosis of a fracture in addition to the extent of injury, and these should all be taken into consideration when deciding on treatment modalities. These factors include the patient's age, bone quality, associated soft tissue injury and other medical conditions. A few social elements to consider include lifestyle, occupation, and hand dominance. Additionally, you should take into account the baseline functional status of the patient. For example, what is their ambulatory ability, assistive devices (cane, walker…), handedness, smoking status etc.

As one gains more experience in the field, it is clear to recognize that there are numerous approaches to managing fractures beyond the simple "surgical vs. nonsurgical." Whenever possible, non-operative treatment is preferred, and this may consist of splinting and casting; these provide semi-rigid immobilization to the broken fragments, thus allowing (secondary) healing with minimal disturbance. **Note:** Acute fractures should generally *not* be casted owing to swelling that can put soft tissue at risk by impairing the circulation. Although non-operative management may seem like a harmless approach, it does not come without its complications. The following are important, potentially disabling

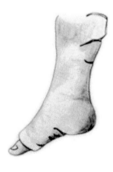

Figure 4: Cast (does not allow for swelling as does a splint)

consequences of improper use of casting or splinting.

- **Pressure necrosis** – An improperly placed cast may cause this as early as 2 hours after its application!
- **Compartment syndrome** – This generally occurs when the compartment pressures *exceed 30 mmHg*. This may be a result from the swelling that occurs after an acute injury. The classic signs and symptoms that may indicate this condition include **the 5 P's (pain, paresthesias, pulselessness, pallor,** and **paralysis)**. *Pain to passive stretch* and a *tense extremity* are very sensitive signs. **Note**: distal pulses may remain present long after muscle and nerve damage are irreversible, and is oftentimes the last to disappear. Also keep in mind that an open fracture does *not* necessarily preclude the development of compartment syndrome, as other fascial compartments may be intact. Compartment syndrome is described in greater detail on page 87.

    Joint stiffness – Prolonged immobilization is a key risk factor, especially for the shoulder and the elbow joints. See "adhesive capsulitis" on page 32.

    Thrombophlebitis – The risk of venous clots is particularly increased with lower extremity fractures and immobilization, as in the elderly after a hip injury

Stress fractures are those caused by repetitive microtrauma, particularly when the amount or intensity of an activity is increased too rapidly. This causes muscles to become fatigued, which eventually transfer the overload to the bone, resulting in a tiny crack. Most stress fractures occur in the weight bearing bones of the lower leg and foot, as in runners who suddenly increase their training. It is important to note that sometimes stress fractures cannot be seen on regular x-rays, or will not show up for several weeks after the pain starts. The most important treatment is to REST the affected bone for 6-8 weeks so as to not engage in activities that reproduce pain (further stress on the fracture may result in a true complete fracture).

Sprains are a very common injury, particularly in athletes but also in the general population. A sprain is when a ligament is overloaded, resulting in its tear (versus a strain, in which a muscle is overstretched resulting in its tear). This occurs when the joint is stretched beyond its normal anatomic barriers. Sprains are GRADED from I to III as follows:

Grade	Physical Exam	Pathophysiology	Typical Treatment
1	Minimal tenderness /swelling	Ligament overstretching → micro tearing	Weight bearing as tolerated Full range-of-motion Stretching/ strengthening exercises RICE
2	Increased joint laxity, Decreased ROM	Partially torn ligament	Immobilization Physical therapy with ROM and stretching/ strengthening exercises
3	Significant swelling, tender, instability, Complete loss of function	Completely ruptured ligament	Immobilization Physical therapy Possible surgery

As various parts of the musculoskeletal are susceptible to local injury, there are also several generalized conditions that are prevalent; one of the most common is **osteoarthritis (OA).** This is a degenerative disease of the joints that results in the progressive loss of articular cartilage. The most common locations for OA are the joints in the hands, hips, and the knees. Joint pain is very vague as there can be several etiologies for this (neurologic, inflammatory, referred pain, traumatic, bursitis etc.). There are several modifiable predisposing factors of osteoarthritis that are important to consider, including obesity, trauma, hard labor, and muscle weakness. These patients will present with deep aching joint pain that is often worse in the morning, joint effusion, decreased range of motion, and stiffness (<60 minutes). This pain is

19

generally exacerbated by exercise. Certain characteristics seen on radiographs can aid in the diagnosis of this condition; 4 particular findings that are important to commit to memory include *joint space narrowing, osteophytes, subchondral sclerosis,* and *subchondral cysts.*

The **Outerbridge classification** is used to assess chondromalacia (softening of articular cartilage as in OA) endoscopically, such as during a diagnostic knee arthroscopy. Types 1-4 correspond to *softening* (Type 1), *fissuring* (Type 2), *"crabmeat" appearance* (Type 3), and *exposed subchondral bone* (Type 4). This is better understood through direct visualization and practice. Laboratory values are generally *normal* in OA, despite the decreased mineralization of the bone. This is important as it helps differentiate osteoarthritis from other diseases that may present similarly. **Note:** this condition differs from Rheumatoid Arthritis, which generally has <u>symmetrical involvement</u>, affects the <u>synovium</u>, and <u>involves the MCP joints</u> of the hand (does not in osteoarthritis). Radiographic findings more specific for rheumatoid arthritis in addition to joint space narrowing include periarticular osteoporosis, ankylosis, and joint erosion. As mentioned before, cancellous bone is the most affected part of the skeleton in OA.

The first line of treatment consists of Acetaminophen, combined with lifestyle modifications and physical therapy. As disease advances and further impairs one's normal daily functions, total joint replacements may be an option.

When considering your list of differential diagnoses (in a patient presenting with any sort of complaint), a useful mnemonic to consider is V.I.N.D.I.C.A.T.E, representing the following causes:
Vascular
Infectious
Neoplasm
Degenerative
Iatrogenic
Congenital
Autoimmune
Trauma
Endocrine

So for example, when a patient presents with non-specific joint pain, there is a long list of potential diagnoses beside osteoarthritis to consider. For example, you can consider hemarthrosis, septic arthritis, sickle cell ischemia, neurologic compression, fibromyalgia, polymyositis, referred hip pain, avascular necrosis, rheumatoid arthritis, bursitis, tendonitis etc...

Additionally, a septic joint is of great concern and requires emergent care. One of the main roles of an orthopedic consult for joint pain is to rule out a septic joint. These patients often have erythema, swelling, and warmth of the joint with or without a fever. Many of them are also unable to bear weight. **A septic joint**, such as of the hip, should be suspected if the patient presents with a fever, non-weight bearing, ESR > 40, and a WBC count > 12,000 This is known as the **Kocher criteria** in pediatrics. The most common cause of a septic joint is *Staphylococcus aureus* in adults or *Neisseria gonorrhoeae* in younger, sexually active adults. Also consider *Propionibacterium acnes* for septic shoulders! It is important to get x-rays to rule out other causes for the physical findings. Remember that plain films are oftentimes negative in the early period (within the first 10 days), and late findings can show joint space narrowing and cartilage destruction. You should also order an ESR/CRP (although nonspecific), WBC count, and blood cultures.

Joint aspiration is the gold standard in diagnosis and a WBC count of the fluid of >50,000 is highly indicative. (Any time you aspirate a joint, you should order a cell (WBC/RBC) count, crystals, gram stain, and culture). In a prosthetic joint that is potentially infected, a WBC count >1500 is the threshold. In this case you also want to consider coagulase-negative staphylococcus. The treatment of choice for a septic joint is generally IV antibiotics, adjusted for the culture and sensitivity of the fluid.

Screws

Being thrown into the discipline, you will hear of various designs and types of screws being mentioned when considering how to manage particular fractures. Therefore, it will certainly help to get a brief understanding of a few of the common types of screws that are used and how they differ from one another. This is a topic that can be discussed extensively, so this brief overview should simplify it to a rather basic level.

Basic screw design is best understood by appreciating certain definitions. The *core diameter* is referred to as the diameter of the solid, central part of the screw from which the threads extend. The *threads* of a screw are the helical ridges that extend outward and essentially clench the bone. **Note**: The core diameter of the screw is how the surgeon determines the size of the drill bit to be used to create the "pilot hole," which is the hole used to guide the screw. It is important to understand that each drill hole represents a site for stress concentration (potential fracture area). The *pitch* is defined as the longitudinal distance between threads. The greater the pitch, the more space between the threads. When a screw becomes tight and is meeting resistance, this is referred to as gaining *purchase*. This has to do with the amount of surface area of the thread that is in contact with the bone. One way to increase this contact is by increasing the difference between the core diameter and the outer diameter. This is better understood by physically feeling the "bite." **Note:** not all screws will have purchase. For example, a "locking screw" simply fastens into its corresponding counterpart without the compressive bite seen with a lag screw (described on the next page).

We already defined the core diameter as the diameter of the solid part of the screw from which the threads extend. The outer diameter is the diameter from the end of one thread to another. The greater the difference between the core and outer diameters, the stronger the fixation as there will be more contact with the bone. An additional way to increase bone-to-screw contact can be done by increasing the number of threads per unit length (using a screw with a lower pitch).

Now that we have defined those terms, a few common types of

screws can be described. **Cortical screws** are screws with a shallow thread, a small pitch, and a large core diameter. Because the core diameter is large, the strength of the screw is also strong and able to handle great stress. These sorts of screws are commonly used to attach plates to bones. **Note**: These screws are always fully threaded throughout the screw (in contrast to cancellous screws which may be "partially threaded"). The best ways to grasp these differences is by getting the opportunity to see and touch the screws. If the opportunity ever arises in the operating room, the scrub technician or even the sales representative will generally be happy to teach you.

As just mentioned, **cancellous screws** can be partially or fully-threaded, each used for different purposes. Cancellous screws have a thinner core diameter than cortical screws (less strength), but have wider, and deeper threads. Since the core diameter is thinner, there is a greater outer-to-core diameter ratio, meaning increased contact and subsequently increased holding power.

You will also hear the term **cannulated screws** being used. These screws have a hollow center. The significance of this is that it can be passed over a guide wire (so the core diameter should be greater than that of a standard screw). These guide wires are used to determine the ideal screw position (via intra-operative fluoroscopy) as well as to maintain reduction of a fracture fragment.

There are also different *techniques* of utilizing screws to manage fractures. One function that is worth understanding is the use of a **lag screw.** This involves placing a screw across a fracture site (must be perpendicular to the fracture line) to cause compression of the fragments. To do this, you need to first reduce the fracture (usually via clamps and forceps). The next step is to drill the holes through which the screw will fasten. This entails using 2 different sizes of drill bits. The *near cortex* should be *over-drilled* (corresponding to the outer diameter of the screw that will be used). The far cortex is drilled to the appropriate screw size (core diameter). This allows the screw to freely enter the near cortex, but when going through the far cortex the threads will bite. This will cause compression over the fracture site, which is further stabilized as the head of the screw is flushed against the near cortex. You may hear the term "countersink" be used to describe the head of the screw being flushed to the bone.

Upper Extremity

Acromioclavicular (AC) separations, commonly known as "shoulder separations," are frequently caused by a fall onto a point on the shoulder causing an upward displacement of the clavicle; this is common in contact sports. There are four AC ligaments (anterior, posterior, superior, inferior), and the deltoid and trapezius muscles blend with the superior ligaments. The superior ligament is the strongest of the four. The AC ligament and the two coracoclavicular ligaments (trapezoid and conoid, of which the conoid is the strongest) provide stability to the particular area. [Refer to an atlas to better visualize the anatomic orientation that provides stability to this joint].

With an AC separation, the deformity is visible on both x-ray and physical exam. The patient should be examined with the upper extremity in a dependent position, which stresses the AC joint and emphasizes the step-off deformity; having the patient hold weights can accentuate this space such as when taking a radiograph. In addition to shoulder series, a Zanca view can be taken to better visualize the distal clavicle. This is done with the beam 10 to 15 degrees cephalad. On physical exam, the clinician may notice a downward sag of the shoulder. If the injury is more severe, an associated coracoclavicular ligament disruption may be present resulting in further clavicle displacement. **Note**: measuring the *coracoclavicular distance* (average of 1.1-1.3 cm) aids in assessing ligament disruption. *Conservative* treatment with a sling is generally satisfactory, reserving surgical intervention for patients with persistent issues. For severe grade injuries or for high-level athletes, coracoclavicular ligament reconstruction may be a viable option (definitely a very interesting case to observe!).

The classification of AC separations is based on the degree and direction of displacement of the distal clavicle, in reference to the coracoclavicular ligaments. These range from Types I –VI. This is termed the **Rockwood grading:**
1. Acromioclavicular ligament *sprain*
2. Acromioclavicular ligament *tear*
3. Acromoioclavicular ligament tear PLUS coracoclavicular ligament tear
4. Grade 3 + *posterior* displacement of distal clavicle

5. Grade 3 + *superior* displacement of distal clavicle
6. Grade 3 + *inferior* displacement of distal clavicle

Although each case is patient-specific, a common general rule for management is as follows: grades 4-6 generally require open reduction and ligament reconstruction, grades 1-3 AC separations can be managed conservatively with a sling and physical therapy.

Around the same location occur **clavicle fractures.** The clavicle is the first bone to ossify (~ 5 weeks gestation), and the last bone to fuse (early to mid-20's). These lesions are quite common, and can be the result of a fall on an outstretched hand or direct blunt trauma. This injury is more commonly seen in children, where they heal very well with minimal intervention.

Majority of the time, the fracture occurs at the *middle third* (80%) of the clavicle, as ligaments bind the distal and proximal thirds. The deforming forces on the injury are secondary to the muscle groups attached. The sternocleidomastoid (SCM) and trapezius muscles displace the medial fragment posterosuperiorly, and the pectoralis major muscle pulls the lateral fragment inferomedially. The patient will classically present with the contralateral hand supporting the weight of the affected arm. Be sure to assess the skin integrity to identify an open fracture, or a possible conversion to an open fraction. Ruling out a pneumothorax or any lung injury from the fracture is also important. Most often clavicle fractures can be treated with a sling or figure-of-eight bandage (studies have not really shown one modality being superior to the other), but in the case of severely displaced fractures, especially of the distal 3rd, ORIF is an option due to the risk of nonunion. Surgical intervention may consist of using a plate or even intramedullary fixation. A careful neurovascular exam should be done to assess for injury to the nearby *subclavian artery* and *brachial plexus*, especially in fractures of the medial 3rd of the clavicle. It is also important to note that if there is a posterior displacement of the medial 3rd in particular, then cardiothoracic surgery should be on board for management. AP films are usually sufficient, looking for *shortening* of the clavicle. Indications for operative management include an open fracture, neurovascular injury, skin tenting, displacement of >100% and shortening of >2cm.

Clavicle fractures are oftentimes classified based on location, displacement, angulation, and the pattern using the **Allman classification groups:**

Group 1: Fracture of middle third of the clavicle. This is the *most common location* in both children and adults, as the proximal and distal ends are secured by ligaments.

Group 2: Fracture of the distal third of the clavicle. This is further classified into 3 types based on the relation of the fracture to the *coracoclavicular (CC)* ligaments.
  a. Distal to the CC ligaments or inter-ligamentous
  b. Medial to the CC ligaments
  c. Involvement of AC joint

Group 3: Fracture of proximal third (~5% of cases). The costoclavicular ligaments usually stabilize this portion. In children and teenagers, this may represent epiphyseal injury. Most brachial plexus injuries are also associated with fractures to this location. This group is further sub-classified based on characteristics of the displacement. Posterior displacement is more serious, and requires operative management along with cardiothoracic surgery consultation.

Glenohumeral dislocations are one of the most commonly encountered joint dislocations in the general population. This is because of the anatomy of the joint is oriented to allow for significant range of motion. It is a common injury in young, athletic patients, and may be associated with labral tears, rotator cuff tears, and fractures. These associated injuries vary according to age (<40 commonly get labral tears and >40 get rotator cuff tears). They usually occur *anteriorly* in nature and are caused by excess external rotation of the arm. Anterior dislocations are characterized by an anterior prominence, posterior sulcus, and inability to internally rotate the arm. Patients hold the arm ABDUCTED and EXTERNALLY rotated. Other associated injuries include *fractures of greater tuberosity* and *axillary nerve injury*, resulting in numbness of the lateral aspect of the deltoid. A simple way to test for axillary nerve function is by testing for the presence of sensation to this area. (The sensory distribution in testing the musculoskeletal nerve will be on the anterolateral aspect of the forearm.) **Note**: *Young patients* have a high incidence of recurrent dislocations (age is actually one of the biggest determinants for this). Consider this: one of the most common complications of a shoulder dislocation is *redislocation.*

Posterior dislocations are uncommon and may occur after massive uncoordinated muscle contractions, as from *seizures* or *electric burns.* In posterior dislocations, patients hold their affected extremity close to the body, but INTERNALLY rotated. On exam one may observe a flattening of the anterior shoulder and a prominent coracoid process. It is commonly missed on standard AP films and requires an *axillary view* to make the diagnosis, as it will show the humeral head posterior to the glenoid cavity, and may also depict a Hill-Sachs lesion (see below). An axillary view is taken with the arm abducted, and the beam directed at the axilla. This view must be ordered! Management involves closed reduction, usually in the emergency department but may need to go to the OR. Technique options include the Milch, Stimson, and Hippocratic maneuvers, and really depend on physician preference. Reduction is followed by immobilization in a sling for around two weeks, along with physical therapy.

As mentioned, regular x-rays may miss posterior dislocations. If evident on radiographs, it may show an internal rotation of the humeral head with a circular appearance *(light bulb sign),* a widened joint space of > 6 mm, or two parallel cortical bone lines on the medial aspect of the humeral head *(trough line sign).*

In addition to the AP and axillary views, a standard shoulder trauma series also includes a "scapular Y" view; this is done with the beam parallel to the scapula, allowing better visualization of the humeral head position. Inferior dislocations of the glenohumeral joint are very rare, and is termed *luxatio erecta.*

Important anatomy
- The shoulder joint has the most range of motion of any joint in the body
- During shoulder abduction, the ratio of glenohumeral joint to scapulothoracic articulation motion is *2 to 1.*
- Glenohumeral ligaments include the superior, middle, and

inferior (none posteriorly or superiorly). The inferior has an anterior and posterior, and these together contribute to shoulder stability

There are specific lesions that may occur resulting in recurrent shoulder instability. A "**HAGL**" injury is a **H**umeral **A**vulsion of the **G**lenohumeral **L**igaments, particularly the *inferior* ligament. This is commonly the result of acute traumatic subluxation. If it is not recognized (essentially unnoticeable on MRI) or repaired, it is associated with a fairly high recurrence rate of dislocations, and may indicate the need for an open repair (opposed to arthroscopic).

A **Bankart lesion** is characterized by an avulsion of the labrum off of the a*nteroinferior* glenoid rim, generally occurring in the setting of shoulder dislocations. The fact that the labrum has a poor blood supply impairs its healing and compromises the stability of the shoulder joint, deeming it susceptible to repeated dislocations. When this is associated with a glenoid rim fracture, it is referred to as a "bony bankart." On examination, pain and clicking with compression and rotation of the shoulder may be elicited, revealing apprehension ("compression test"). A combination of x-ray (*West point view* – patient prone, beam directed at axilla to depict anterior inferior glenoid, 25 degrees cephalad and 25 degrees medial), MRI, and arthrogram supplemented with a keen suspicion are required for a diagnosis. These lesions can be managed arthroscopically or open.

Another complication of glenohumeral dislocations (and bankart lesions) is termed a **Hill-Sachs lesion.** This is a defect on the *posterolateral* head of the humerus caused by chondral impaction on the glenoid. The impression fracture on the humerus is at risk of enlarging and further compromising the glenohumeral joint. This is most commonly seen with *repeated* anterior dislocations. If the defect causes the joint to move abnormally, it is termed "engaging," and usually requires additional surgical treatment. A special *Hill-Sach view* is used to visualize the posterolateral defect; it is an AP radiograph taken with the shoulder in maximal internal rotation. Treatment options consist of conservative management, a capsular shift, bone grafting, disimpaction, or a total shoulder replacement (indicated only in elderly patients).

The **Rotator Cuff** of the shoulder consists of the muscles that provide stability to the shoulder joint and can demonstrate varying pathology including impingement, tendonitis, and tears. It consist of the supraspinatus, infraspinatus, teres minor, and subscapularis muscles [Mnemonic: **SITS**]. The *supraspinatus* is the most commonly torn tendon due to its susceptibility to impingement as it runs inferior to the acromion. This is commonly seen in throwers or people with repeated overhead activities. These patients will generally present with pain with overhead movement and pain at night that wakes them up from sleep. Radiograph may show calcium deposition of the tendons (calcific tendonitis), along with spurs depending on its chronicity. Humeral head elevation may occur as one of the functions of the rotator cuff is to prevent this, and this may potentiate arthritis. This may be evident on plain radiographs. MRI *with contrast* is particularly helpful in depicting the communication between the joint and the subacromial space, as well as fatty infiltration. The **Goutallier classification** can be used on MRI to determine whether surgical intervention would be beneficial. This assesses cuff atrophy based on fat infiltration of the tendon; when a tendon ruptures, depending on the severity and chronicity, it may retract significantly off of its attachment and become reversibly infiltrated with fat. The Goutallier classification goes as follows:

> **Grade 1** - fatty streaks
> **Grade 2** - fat < muscle
> **Grade 3** - fat = muscle
> **Grade 4** - fat > muscle

If conservative management does not help, then operative management with subacromial decompression or total rotator cuff repair with anchors are options depending on the patient. Remember that in addition to the pathology, you have to take into consideration the functional status and goals of the patient. What is the patient's baseline? What is the handedness of the patient? What does he/she expect to be doing with the fixed arm? Shoulder replacements are indicated in older patients (usually over the age of 70), who have atrophied rotator cuff muscles. The "reverse" total shoulder replacement is a procedure that is becoming more and more common, and has positive outcomes. The concept behind this is to utilize the deltoid as the main arm flexor/abductor since the rotator cuff is atrophied and its functional use is impaired.

Normally, the shoulder is a ball-and-socket joint with the proximal humerus being the ball and the glenoid being the socket. In a reverse total shoulder, a prosthesis is placed in where the proximal humerus becomes the "socket" and the glenoid becomes the "ball" part of the joint. **Note**: to perform this procedure the patient must have a functional deltoid muscle, and this requires that the axillary nerve be intact (assess sensation to the lateral shoulder).

In addition to the standard palpation, range of motion, and neurovascular exam as a part of the physical exam of the shoulder, several specific rotator cuff tests should be considered to aid in a diagnosis (watching videos will help better visualize these):

- **Jobe's empty can test**
  - Assesses the strength and integrity of the *supraspinatus*
    - Abduct the shoulder 90 degrees and anteriorly on a horizontal plane ~30 degrees
    - Thumbs point down (like pouring a can of soda)
    - Apply downward force to the patient's forearm
    - Assess for pain or decreased strength
- **External rotation**
  - Assesses *infraspinatus* and *teres minor*
    - With elbow flexed at 90 degrees and externally rotated 45 degrees, assess resistance to internal rotation
    - Significant infraspinatus weakness may indicate injury to *suprascapular* nerve (trauma, ganglion cyst etc.)
- **Lift-off test**
  - Assesses *subscapularis*
  - Have patient internally rotate arm behind their back, with the dorsum of the hand on the lower back
  - Ask patient to lift back of hand off of lower back
  - Inability to lift off suggests a positive finding

- **Neer's impingement**
  - Impingement of rotator cuff, particularly *supraspinatus* under subacromial arch
  - Stabilize scapula with one hand
  - Passively flex the patient's arm with the other hand
  - Assess for pain in anterior shoulder or reproduction of symptoms

- **Hawkin-Kennedy impingement**
  - Assess rotator cuff impingement
  - Arm flexed to 90 degrees
  - Elbow bent to 90 degrees on horizontal plane
  - Holding proximal to the elbow, use the other arm to internally rotate patient's elbow
  - Assess for pain in anterior shoulder or reproduction of symptoms
- **Load and shift test**
  - Assess shoulder stability in anterior-posterior planes
  - With patient seated or supine, grasp anterior head of the humerus and apply anterior-posterior glide from its resting position
  - Positive test is suggested by excessive gliding, which can be graded on a scale of 1-3
- **Apprehension test**
  - Assesses anterior stability
  - With patients arm abducted to 90 degrees and elbow flexed 90, provide a posterior to anterior force at the head of the humerus
  - Pain or fear of dislocation suggests a positive test
- **O'brien's test**

SLAP - superior labrum from anterior to posterior. The **Crank test** can also be used, which is abducting the arm, axial compression, and rotation. An arthrogram is the most sensitive for labral tears.

  - Assesses integrity of glenoid labrum (***SLAP* tear**) and acromioclavicular joint
  - Patient is instructed to flex shoulder to 90 degrees, adduct ~ 15 degrees, internally rotate arm with thumb facing down
  - Apply downward force
  - Then instruct patient to externally rotate arm with thumbs toward ceiling, and again apply a downward force

32

- o Pain or popping in the internally rotated but not externally rotated position is considered positive
- o **Note**: A higher grade injury involves a tear of the bicipital tendon (where it anchors to the labrum), and so the Speed Test may also be positive. The Speed Test assesses for bicipital tendon pathology and is done by having the patient flex their arm against resistance, with the arm extended, and forearm supinated.
- o SLAP lesions are important to grade as the severity affects management.
  - Type 1 tear is defined by labral fraying
  - Type 2 has a labrum that is *detached*
  - Type 3 tear is *bucket handle* in nature
  - Type 4 is a bucket handle lesion PLUS associated detachment of the biceps

Although not a hard and fast rule, a general rule of thumb is that types 2 and 4 can be repaired, whereas types 1 and 3 should be debrided.

Important anatomy

- The trapezius and serratus anterior muscles are related to the shoulder, and if weakened result in *lateral* and *medial* winging of the scapula, respectively.
- A fracture to the anatomic neck of the humerus increases the risk of *osteonecrosis*. The posterior humeral circumflex artery (off of the axillary artery) is one of the main vessels supplying the femoral head.
- A fracture to the surgical neck is common, particularly in the elderly.
- The greater tuberosity is the insertion site of *supraspinatus, infraspinatus, teres minor*.
- The lesser tuberosity is the insertion site of *subscapularis*.
- The **rotator interval** is the space between the tendons of the supraspinatus and the subscapularis. It consists of the *superior glenohumeral ligament* and the *coracohumeral ligament*. The long head of the biceps tendon also contributes to stability to this area.

Adhesive capsulitis ("frozen shoulder") is defined as pain and stiffness of the shoulder secondary to synovial inflammation and capsular fibrosis. This ultimately leads to adhesions and a contracted capsule. This is common after prolonged immobilization of the shoulder, but is also associated with medical conditions as diabetes and thyroid disorders. On exam, the patient will have a decrease in *both* active and passive range of motion, especially with *external rotation*. Patients may also complain of the <u>pain waking them up at night</u>. As x-rays are generally normal, an MR arthrogram may show a *loss of the axillary recess,* indicating contracture of the joint capsule. Management is usually conservative with NSAIDs, PT, and steroid injections. A failure to improve may indicate arthroscopic lysis of adhesions, or manipulation under sedation. Manipulation is essentially moving the extremity through the restricted ranges of motion by tearing the adhesions. Complications of adhesive capsulitis include axillary nerve injury, rotator cuff tendon disruption, and recurrent stiffness.

The most common fracture of the humerus would be a **proximal humerus fracture,** often seen in the *elderly* population secondary to osteoporosis (remember, cancellous bone is most susceptible) and trauma. The major blood supply to this area is from the anterior and posterior humeral circumflex arteries, branching off of the axillary artery. As the *axillary nerve* courses just anteroinferior to the glenohumeral joint, it is particularly susceptible to injury in a proximal humerus fracture. Do you remember how the sensory aspect of the nerve is tested on physical exam? Motor testing is often not possible secondary to pain. Patients typically present with the affected extremity held close to the chest, supported by the contralateral hand.

Proximal humerus fractures can be classified using the **Neer classification**, which is based on the number of fragment parts. A fragment is defined as a "part" if there is > 1cm of displacement or 45 degrees of angulation. The exception is the greater tuberosity, which has a tolerance of 5mm displacement. The reason for this exception is two-fold. Firstly, the rotator cuff muscles attach there so there may be resultant dysfunction. Secondly, the displacement can result in subacromial impingement.
- The 4 parts consist of the femoral head, greater tuberosity,

lesser tuberosity, and humeral shaft. Several combinations of fragments are possible.

- One-part fracture: no displaced fragments regardless of number of fracture lines
- Two-part fracture: Fracture of either the anatomic neck, surgical neck, greater tuberosity, or lesser tuberosity.
- Three-part fracture: Surgical neck fracture AND either the greater or lesser tuberosity.

If no fragments are displaced, then the fracture is considered stable, which is the most common presentation. This is treated with immobilization via sling and early exercise. Avascular necrosis is a potential complication, especially with fractures of the anatomic neck. Fortunately, proximal fractures in children have excellent remodeling potential.

Important anatomical considerations:

- Supraspinatus and external rotators displace the greater tuberosity superiorly
- The subscapularis displaces the lesser tuberosity medially
- The pectoralis major displaces the humeral shaft medially
- The deltoid abducts the proximal humerus

Humeral shaft fractures present with pain and deformity around the mid-humeral region, most commonly secondary to trauma. The displacement is based on the deforming forces of the muscles along with the location of the fracture. The primary deforming forces are from the *pectoralis* and *deltoid* muscles. *Radial nerve palsy* is often associated with this type of injury due to the fact that the nerve runs on the surface of the bone (in the *spiral groove*). Study your anatomy! Most humeral fractures will heal with nonsurgical management such as closed reduction and splinting. Important acceptable tolerances that will not compromise function or appearance are as follows:

- **20 degrees anterior-posterior angulation**
- **30 degrees varus-valgus angulation**
- **3 cm shortening**

A spiral fracture involving the distal 1/3 of the radius in adults may cause entrapment of the radial nerve, and is termed a **Holstein-Lewis fracture**. This results in dysfunction of the innervations distal to the injury (extensor muscles of forearm and wrist), presenting as "wrist drop." Both neuropraxia and axonotmesis may result. For an open fracture, debridement of the wound, exploration of the nerve and fixation of the fracture should be done. An *anterolateral* approach should be used, exploring the nerve between the brachialis and brachioradialis muscles. **Note:** radial nerve palsy is not a contraindication to functional bracing, as the palsy may be (and often is) transient. Also remember that a spiral fracture in the long bone of a child is generally from a high-energy force, possibly secondary to abuse.

Second to shoulder dislocations come **elbow dislocations**, most commonly *posterior* in nature, and most commonly in the 10 to 20-year-old population. The mechanism is usually a combination of supination of the forearm, along with a valgus force. This may happen from a fall on an outstretched hand resulting in the olecranon unlocking from the trochlea. The LCL fails first, and then depending on the degree of injury, the MCL. The capsuloligamentous injury progresses from *lateral to medial* and is termed the *Hori Circle*. Associated injuries include complex fractures, which can present as the **"terrible triad"** –a radial head fracture, and a coronoid fracture, and an elbow dislocation. On x-ray, the *fat pad sign* may be seen (also known as the "sail sign"). This is secondary to displacement of the fat pad around the elbow joint (by an effusion) from an intra-articular fracture.

Important anatomy
- The elbow really consists of 3 joints (proximal radioulnar joint, radiohumeral joint, and ulnohumeral joint)
- Acute neurovascular compromise is uncommon, but when it does occur affects *the ulnar nerve, anterior interosseus nerve, or brachial artery.*
- The *anterior bundle* of the medial collateral ligament is the most important restraint to valgus stress. It attaches to the *"sublime tubercle"* of the coronoid process. Its strength is demonstrated by the fact that the elbow can completely

dislocate with this anterior bundle remaining intact.

A very common overuse injury of the elbow is **lateral epicondylitis,** oftentimes referred to as "tennis elbow." This occurs secondary to repetitive wrist extension, ultimately resulting in tendinosis and inflammation of the common extensor tendons as they insert on the lateral epicondyle (most commonly affected is the *extensor carpi radialis brevis* [ecrb]*)*. Patients present with point tenderness to the lateral elbow, particularly at the insertion of the ECRB, and pain with gripping activities. Provocative tests can help in diagnosing this, such as resisted wrist extension, or maximal passive flexion reproducing the pain. As the diagnosis is mostly clinical, radiographs are recommended only to rule out other causes. First line of treatment consists of activity modification, RICE, NSAIDs, and physical therapy. There are various braces and straps that can aid some patients. Steroid injections are also an option. If nonoperative management fails after a year, operative release and debridement of the ECRB origin may resolve the problem. As this is not the main wrist extensor, and other muscles such as the extensor carpi ulnaris will still be intact, wrist extension will be minimally affected by this procedure. The corresponding overuse injury of the medial epicondyle is termed "golfer's elbow."

Important anatomy
- Extensor tendons attach on the *lateral* epicondyle
    - Anconeus
    - Supinator
    - Extensor carpi radialis brevis
    - Extensor carpi ulnaris
    - Extensor digiti minimi
    - Extensor digitorum
- Flexor tendons attach on the *medial epicondyle*
    - Pronator teres
    - Palmaris longus
    - Flexor carpi radialis
    - Flexor carpi ulnaris
    - Flexor digitorum superficialis
    - Flexor pollicis longus

Ulnar shaft fractures may be described specifically by the location and any associated lesions in the area. For example, a ***Monteggia lesion*** (Figure 5) is defined as a fracture of the proximal ulna with an associated radial head dislocation. As Monteggia lesions can occur via several mechanisms, the **Bado classification** system categorizes it into four types, based on the direction of radial head displacement:

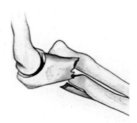

Type I: Anterior (most common)
Type II: Posterior
Type III: Lateral
Type IV: Anterior with associated radial head fracture

Figure 5: Monteggia lesion

These patients present with elbow swelling, deformity, and painful range of motion. It is crucial to assess the compartments for the complication of compartment syndrome, along with evaluating the wrist and elbow, *especially the distal radioulnar joint.*

Almost three times as common as Monteggia fractures are **Galeazzi fractures** (Figure 6). These fractures are defined as those of the distal third of the radius with an associated disruption of the distal radioulnar joint (DRUJ). Other names for this type of injury are

A *reverse Galeazzi* refers to a fracture of the distal ulna with associated distal radioulnar joint dislocation

"fracture of necessity" (since it requires ORIF) and a Piedmont fracture. Similar to the

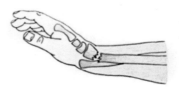

Monteggia, it is important to check the compartments and assess the wrist and elbow. The recommended operative approach is termed an anterior Henry approach, which is between the flexor carpi radialis and the brachioradialis. Understand the internervous planes both proximally and distally (radial and median nerves).

Figure 6: Galeazzi lesion

Among the most common fractures of the upper extremity are those of the **distal radius**. The incidence of these fractures rises with increasing age. Guaranteed to see in every emergency department! The elderly are particularly susceptible due to osteoporosis, and these lesions can be predictors for future

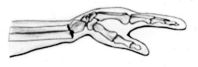

Figure 8: Colles fx

fractures (DEXA scans are recommended). 80% of axial load is supported by the distal radius, along with numerous ligamentous attachments. Interestingly, these ligaments often remain intact in such fractures, allowing adequate reduction through "ligamentotaxis." The wrist is typically swollen/deformed with ecchymosis, tenderness, and painful range of motion. A careful neurovascular assessment should be performed with particular attention to *median nerve function.* Of course, there are eponyms for all the variations of distal radius fractures. **Colles fractures (comprising >90% of distal radius fx)** *are dorsally* displaced and described as "dinner fork deformities" due to its appearance on lateral film with *volar angulation* (Figure 7). The mechanism is a fall onto a hyperextended, radially deviated wrist with the forearm in pronation. In contrast, the **Smith fracture** (Figure 8) is sustained by a fall onto a flexed wrist with the

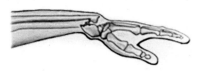

Figure 7: Smith fx (apex dorsal, volar angulation)

forearm in supination. This results in a *volar* displaced fracture. This is an *unstable* fracture pattern and usually requires surgical intervention. **Barton's fracture** is an intra-articular fracture with dislocation of the radiocarpal joint. *Carpal displacement along with displacement of the rim of the radius* is what distinguishes this fracture. (A volar barton's is more common than a dorsal Barton's). A **Chauffeur's fracture** is an avulsion of the styloid process of the radius with extrinsic ligaments remaining attached; it also referred to as a "backfire fracture" or a "Hutchinson fracture."

The commonly used **Frykman classification** for Colles' fractures is based on the pattern of joint involvement (radiocarpal and/or radioulnar +/- ulnar styloid fracture). Although it does not necessarily guide management, it is a good classification system to understand, and is defined as the following types:

1,2: Extraarticular
3,4: radiocarpal joint involved
5,6: radioulnar joint involved
7,8: both radiocarpal & radioulnar joints
[even numbered types have an associated ulnar styloid fracture]

On radiographic evaluation, certain <u>normal</u> values should be kept in mind to assess the injury:

Radial inclination: ~ 23 degrees
Radial height: ~ 11 mm
Volar tilt: ~ 12 degrees
[Mnemonic: (11 + 12 = 23)]

Importantly, all displaced fractures should undergo closed reduction regardless of future surgical management. This helps to limit post injury swelling, provides pain relief, and relieves compression of the median nerve. Usually the fracture can be reduced under a "hematoma block," which is an injection of anesthetic into a peri-fracture hematoma. As you will see in the emergency room, a common way to reduce these fractures is by suspending the hand by two fingers, with the elbow flexed to 90 degrees. The traction from gravity oftentimes brings these injuries out to length with only minor adjustments required by the practitioner. This is particularly beneficial in the elderly as manipulating the deformity with strength is not as necessary as it may be in children. Some fractures will re-displace following closed manipulation; the propensity for re-displacement depends on both the *initial degree of displacement* and the *age* of the patient.

The greatest influence on outcome following a distal radius fracture is *carpal alignment*. This is measured by the intersection of two lines on a lateral radiograph; one line is drawn parallel through the middle of the radial shaft, and the other through and parallel to the capitate. If the two lines intersect within the wrist, then the carpus is aligned. As for treatment options, there are several and include closed reduction and cast immobilization, external fixation, ORIF, and *percutaneous pinning*.

> **Complications**:
> Poor grip strength
> Median nerve injury
> Malunion or nonunion (painful or painless)
> Reflex sympathetic dystrophy
> Post-traumatic osteoarthritis

Radial head fractures commonly occur with associated fractures or ligamentous injuries to other parts of the same extremity. *Make sure you check the stability of the distal radioulnar joint!* The most common fracture site is the *anterolateral portion* of the radial head as it is particularly weak. A commonly utilized classification system is the **Mason Classification,** organized as follows:
1. Nondisplaced
2. Single displaced fragment
3. Comminuted fracture
4. Fracture with associated elbow dislocation

Carpal tunnel syndrome is a potentially disabling condition of the upper extremity that is increasing in prevalence. This problem is often caused by repetitive wrist movements, and results in swelling of the contents of the carpal tunnel. <u>Contents</u> of the tunnel (under the flexor retinaculum) include *the median nerve, flexor digitorum profundus tendons, flexor digitorum superficialis tendons, and the flexor pollicis longus tendon.* Often blamed on overuse mechanisms, carpal tunnel syndrome can also be associated with metabolic conditions including diabetes, amyloidosis, normal pregnancy and thyroid disease. The resulting increase in pressure on the median nerve causes the patient to complain of pain and paresthesias in the nerve's distribution (know it's motor and sensory innervations!) In severe, more chronic cases cases, there can be subsequent wasting of the thenar musculature. The diagnosis is made clinically by eliciting a proper history, such as noting that the symptoms *wake the patient at night* and there is numbness and tingling in the median nerve distribution. In addition to examining

41

the sensory and motor deficits, a Tinel's test and Phalen's tests can be performed. *Tinel's test* involves tapping with a finger over the median nerve just distal to the wrist. This test may be performed for any suspected compressive neuropathy, such as that of the ulnar nerve near the medial elbow. A positive test is indicated by reproduction of the symptoms of pain and paresthesias. *Phalen's test* involves holding the dorsum of the wrists against each other in maximum flexion for 60 seconds, and again observing for any increase or reproduction of symptoms. The more recent *Durkin's compression test* can be used, which is done by using your thumb to put pressure directly over the carpal tunnel for 30 seconds to reproduce symptoms. This is considered the <u>most sensitive</u> test for carpal tunnel.

Conservative treatment consists of NSAIDS, a night splint, and activity modification. Steroid injections are also an option, but relief is generally only for a few months duration. Operative treatment involves cutting the transverse carpal ligament (can be done open or arthroscopically). As this is a common disorder, it is recommended to understand the surgical approach and any surrounding relevant anatomy for the procedure.

DeQuervain's tenosynovitis is a disorder commonly seen in new mothers from repeatedly lifting their children, or other individuals who may have a similar repetitive motion. This essentially results in an inflammation of the tendon sheath overlying the radial styloid process (*First* dorsal compartment). The involved tendons are the *extensor pollicis brevis* and *abductor pollicis longus*. The presentation is generally with pain over the radial side of the wrist, which radiates distally into the thumb. A provocation test to aid in diagnosis is called *Finkelstein's test*. This involves clenching the thumb into the palm of a closed fist, and then ulnar deviating the wrist. A positive test is expressed by tenderness over the 1st dorsal compartment with reproduction of symptoms, and is essentially diagnostic. Conservative treatment includes rest, NSAIDS, and splinting of the thumb. Steroid injections can also be added to the therapy. When non-operative management fails, surgical intervention is used to release the tendon sheath.

Important anatomy

- An entity that may present similarly to DeQuervian's is when there is compression or trauma to a proximal nerve. The superficial radial nerve may become entrapped resulting in similar sensory symptoms, referred to as *cheiralgia paresthetica.* Paresthesia is usually around the anatomical snuffbox. This is differentiated from DeQuervian's since the symptoms are not dependent on motion of the hands or fingers.

Infective tenosynovitis is a finger condition you may encounter as a consult in the Emergency Department. There are 4 particular signs, termed the *Kanavel cardinal signs,* that will indicate the presence of infectious tenosynovitis of the flexor tendon sheaths. These include:

1. Pain with extension of digit
2. Passive flexion of the digit
3. Fusiform (sausage-like) swelling
4. Tenderness over the tendon sheath

Dupuytren contracture is a tightening of the palmar fascia, which draws the finger(s) into flexion. This condition is seen in people with varying risk factors, but two notable ones are *alcoholics* and *rock climbers.* Some patients may have no risk factors. The most commonly involved finger is the ring finger, although fascial nodules can present anywhere on the palm. Palpating nodules in the palm, and noticing that the fingers are unable to be completely extended makes a diagnosis. Conservative treatment involves stretching the fascia in an attempt to prevent further contracture. Surgical excision of the palmar fascia is also an option, but it has complications of injury to the digital nerves that may be entangled in the fascia, and may also recur.

A **Boxer's fracture** is typically caused by punching something (like a wall or a person) and causes a fracture involving the 5th metacarpal neck. The apex of angulation is usually *dorsal.* The particular location for an injury is well tolerated in the sense that even if it heals with 45 degrees of angulation, there is little functional disability. This is in contrast to fractures of the metacarpal shaft that have a lower tolerance. There are different accepted tolerances you may encounter for metacarpal fractures based on different studies. The tolerances for metacarpal shaft fractures are around 10-20-30-40, relating to fingers 2-3-4-5. Most importantly you must understand that the acceptable angulation of deformity increases the more ulnar the injury is. The tolerances for metacarpal neck fractures (from fingers 2-5) are around 10-15-30-45 degrees. Treatment is with reduction followed by an ulnar gutter splint to correct the angulation.

Regarding injuries to the wrist, the bone that is most frequently injured is the scaphoid bone. **Scaphoid fractures** are potentially dangerous due to the tenuous blood supply, making it susceptible to *avascular necrosis* and *nonunion*. The blood supply is from the *dorsal carpal branch, off of the radial artery*, which runs retrograde from distal to proximal. Usually caused by a fall on an outstretched hand, it presents with wrist pain and tenderness in the "anatomic snuffbox." The danger is that minimally displaced fractures of the scaphoid waist are often not visible on a standard AP and lateral x-ray, and so the diagnosis may be missed. If misdiagnosed as a wrist sprain the fracture often goes on to initiate the development of eventual wrist arthritis. For this reason, *scaphoid views* (30 degree wrist extension, 20 degree *ulnar deviation*) are important to consider when ordering radiographs. Due to the fact that radiographs may show false negatives, treatment recommendations suggest that all wrist injuries with tenderness to the anatomic snuffbox be splinted for two weeks, then re-imaged for better clarification. For a nondisplaced fracture, long arm thumb spica casting for 2-4 months is usually successful. But if displaced, then operative treatment is indicated due to the complications mentioned earlier.

Important Anatomy
- The anatomical snuff box is made of the tendons of the *extensor pollicis longus, extensor pollicis brevis*, and *abductor pollicis*

The second most commonly fractured wrist bone is the **triquetrum**. These fractures are commonly avulsion or impaction lesions, and are usually seen on lateral and oblique radiographs.

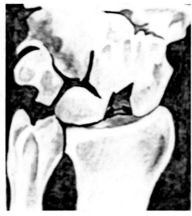

Figure 9: Terry Thomas sign

Another injury caused from falling on an outstretched hand is a **perilunate dislocation.** This is when the carpus is dislocated relative to the lunate, which is in normal alignment with the distal radius. The danger lies in that many physicians have trouble recognizing displacements of the carpal bones. (You should learn to recognize abnormalities of the lunate and look for widening of the space of the surrounding joints, especially the scapho-lunate interval). A scapholunate gap greater than *3mm* is a significant finding on x-ray; this is termed the **Terry Thomas sign** (Figure 9). The weak spot where this dislocation occurs (due to a lack of ligamentous stability) is termed the *Space of Poirier.* Complications include a high risk of median nerve palsy, compartment syndrome, and long-term wrist dysfunction. Therefore treatment warrants prompt open reduction with ligamentous repair if closed reduction is unsuccessful. Note: These are not easy reductions. There is a pattern of injury that occurs in such dislocations termed the *Mayfield instability pattern.* This starts with disruption of the scapholunate joint, then proceeds to the lunocapitate, then the lunotriquetrum, and finally results in a perilunate dislocation.

Do not confuse this with lunate **dislocations**, which are characterized by volar displacement of the lunate *with abnormal radiolunate articulation.* The key to not confusing the two is the *lateral* projection film, in which you see that
>1). Lunate dislocations show radiolunate disruption and volar dislocation
>2). Perilunate dislocations maintain radiolunate articulation

When the thumb is injured, it is important to differentiate between intra- and extra-articular fractures, particularly when the metacarpal base is involved. Carpometacarpal arthritis is one of the most common areas for arthritis in the body. Intra-articular fractures are further broken down into Type I and Type II:

> **Type I (Bennett fracture)**: The fracture line produces a disruption of the first carpometacarpal joint; this results in the metacarpal being pulled proximally/laterally by *the abductor pollicis longus* muscle. This lesion is best seen with the hyper-pronated thumb view.

> **Type II (Rolando fracture)**: Involves a greater force than a Bennett and is described as a comminuted, intra-articular fracture. These have a propensity to cause degenerative joint disease.

Trauma to the thumb may also lead to thumb metacarpophalangeal (MCP) dislocations, which are associated with a torn ulnar collateral ligament. Of particular importance is the **Stener lesion**; this is when the ruptured part of the ulnar collateral ligament becomes entrapped in the adductor pollicis muscle. Clinically this causes a tender prominence that may be seen around the medial base of the thumb.

Ulnar collateral thumb ligament injuries have been described as "Gamekeeper's thumb", based on the historical method of wringing birds' necks. The mechanism of this injury is hyperabduction or extension at the MCP joint of the thumb resulting in a sprain of the ulnar collateral ligament; this is common in skiing accidents where the thumb catches on the strap and is forcefully radially deviated. On exam there may be a mass from a torn ligament and a possible bony avulsion (Stener lesion as described above). There is usually tenderness over the 1st MCP joint and laxity with stress of the ulnar collateral ligament. A lack of pain with stress may be concerning for a completely torn ligament (type 3). For partial tears, immobilization may be the therapy of choice, otherwise ligament repair or reconstruction with tendon grafts are options.

Hand lesions are also a common occurrence varying from lacerations to fractures to masses. One of the most common complaints for a mass or lump in the hand tends to be **Ganglion cysts.** These are synovial fluid-filled cysts arising from a wrist joint. The presenting age is commonly in the younger population, from 15 to 40 years of age. In most cases they are harmless, and tend to develop on the dorsum of the wrist. These cysts are fluid-filled, and can alter quite quickly (they can appear, disappear, grow, shrink). They also *transilluminate*, which can aid in the diagnosis. Unless the cyst is painful or interferes with function, treatment is not needed. Considering they have a tendency to grow with activity, immobilization is one of the therapies, ideally shrinking it. Another option would be aspiration of the cyst. If all else fails, surgery can be performed, but there still remains the chance of recurrence, so it is important to excise the stalk as well.

Lipomas are the most common nonmalignant masses found around the body. They are usually subcutaneous in location, and outside of the fascia, but can occur in deeper tissues as well. Treatment of such lesions is not necessary except to confirm the diagnosis, for cosmetic reasons, or if pain is present.

Lower Extremity

It is important to completely understand the neurovascular distribution pattern of the lower extremity when assessing a patient, particularly for documentation purposes and effective communication. For example, after a lower extremity procedure (i.e. cephalomedullary nail for a subtrochanteric fracture), it is key to test motor and sensory function distal to the area that was treated. Total hip and knee arthroplasties are also extremely common these days so it is significant. So know for example that L3 nerve root represents the function of the quadriceps, L4 for the tibialis anterior, L5 for the extensor hallucis longus, and S1 with the gastrocnemius/soleus. This can be documented simply as motor function of L3-S1 nerve roots. Knowing the sensory innervation for each of these nerve roots is also essential, such as the fact that the deep peroneal nerve innervates the web space between the first and second toes. On examination, pulses should be checked at the dorsalis pedis, posterior tibial, and popliteal arteries whenever possible.

Additionally, it is important to know the different compartments of the leg, as this can be particularly significant when suspecting compartment syndrome. The leg has 4 compartments: lateral, anterior, superficial posterior, and deep posterior. Understand the contents of each compartment. Note: You should do the same for the compartments of the hand, the forearm, the arm, and the thigh, as compartment syndrome can occur in any of these locations.

Hip dislocations are frequent reasons for orthopedic consults in the emergency room, and also constitute an orthopedic emergency. Most commonly, these are posterior in nature (~90%) and result from impaction of the knee on the dashboard, as in unrestrained motorists. (**Anterior dislocations** result *from external rotation and abduction of* the hip). The direction ultimately is determined by the direction of the pathologic force, and the position of the extremity at the time of injury. For patients with hip dislocations, up to 50% sustain concomitant fractures elsewhere as it is generally from a trauma. Two important consequences of hip dislocations are *femoral head osteonecrosis* and *sciatic nerve injury.*

Another situation where posterior hip dislocations are of particular importance are in patients who have had total hip replacements. This specifically holds true if a posterior approach to the hip was used, as in this approach the short external rotators are generally weakened because they are cut to provide access to the capsule.

With pelvic fractures, a full trauma survey is essential because of the high-energy nature of these injuries. The classic appearance of a patient with a posterior dislocation is with the hip in **_flexion, internal rotation,_** and **_adduction._** (Patients with anterior dislocations hold the hip in marked external rotation). In posterior dislocations, the **sciatic nerve** may be injured (presenting more commonly as an isolated peroneal portion of the nerve with foot drop). Rarely, injury to the femoral neurovascular structures may occur as a result from an anterior dislocation.

In regards to radiographic evaluation, obtain AP and lateral films of the hip as well as an AP pelvis. In posterior dislocations, the affected femoral head will appear smaller than the normal femoral head. In contrast, in anterior dislocations the femoral head may appear larger. _Shenton's line_ (Figure 10) is an imaginary line drawn along the inferior border of the superior pubic ramus and along the inferomedial border of the femoral neck. This line should be smooth and continuous, otherwise indicating a possible associated fracture/displacement of the femoral neck. Femoral neck

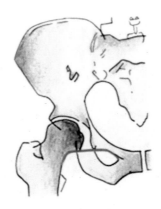

Figure 10: Shenton's line

fractures are more common with anterior dislocations. It is also important to mention that if a prosthetic hip is noted on radiograph, then the clinician should carefully assess for _periprosthetic fractures_ and _loosening_ of hardware.

Classification of hip dislocations is based on the relationship of the femoral head to the acetabulum, and the presence of any associated fractures. Posterior hip dislocations are classified using the

49

Thompson classification system:
1. No or minor posterior wall fracture of acetabulum
2. Large posterior wall fracture
3. Comminuted acetabular fracture
4. Acetabular floor fracture
5. Femoral head fracture

Urgent reduction should ensue to minimize the risk of avascular necrosis of the femoral head, ideally *within 6 hours.* The long-term prognosis worsens if reduction is delayed for more than 12 hours. Keep in mind that the complication of osteonecrosis may become clinically apparent *years* after injury. A factor that may contribute to this vascular complication is repeated attempts at reduction, so limiting the number of attempts in the ED is also important.

Reducing the hip can be done with numerous techniques, but usually requires heavy sedation and physical effort by the physician; general anesthesia with paralysis in the operating room may even be necessary. Make sure to get post-reduction films and repeat the neurovascular exam! These patients should also be put on "hip precautions." This means they should be restricted from extreme hip flexion, adduction, internal rotation for 6 weeks post-reduction to prevent the risk of re-dislocation. The most frequent long-term complication of hip dislocations is posttraumatic osteoarthritis. *Sciatic nerve injuries* are a complication as mentioned earlier, occurring from stretching of the nerve by a posteriorly dislocated hip. EMG studies may be indicated at 3-4 weeks for baseline information and prognostic guidance.

Important anatomy
- The acetabulum is formed by confluence of the ischium, ilium, and pubis bones.
- 40% of the femoral head is covered by the acetabulum at any position. The labrum deepens the acetabulum and increases stability of the joint.
- The main vascular supply to the femoral head is from the medial and lateral femoral circumflex, branches of the deep (profunda) femoral artery. The most significant of the medial circumflex is the *lateral epiphyseal branch.* Occasionally, the artery of the ligamentum teres/foveal artery (branch of obturator artery) may contribute to the

supply. This is of greater importance in the pediatric population.

- The sciatic nerve exits the pelvis at the greater sciatic notch (along with several other structures which are important to know).
- Muscles that insert on the greater trochanter are the *piriformis, gluteus medius, gluteus minimus, obturator internus,* and *superior gemellus.*

Femoral head fractures are almost always associated with concomitant hip dislocations. As these are commonly from high-energy injuries, a formal trauma evaluation is generally necessary. Understanding the anatomy of the femoral head is important in classifying the fractures, as this affects management. The fovea capitis of the femoral head is the portion that has no cartilage, and is where the ligamentum teres attaches. Through this ligament runs the foveal artery that contributes to the blood supply to the head. The classification system used is the **Pipkin classification.** This is broken down into 4 types as follows:

1. Hip dislocation with fracture *inferior* to fovea capitis
2. Hip dislocation with fracture *superior* to fovea capitis
3. Type 1 or 2 with *associated femoral neck fracture*
4. Type 1 or 3 with *associated acetabular rim fracture*

One of the most commonly encountered orthopedic injuries, particularly in the elderly population, are hip fractures. These can be defined as femoral neck fractures, intertrochanteric fractures, or subtrochanteric fractures. Each of these will be explained below.

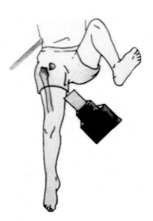

Femoral neck fractures are important injuries to manage expeditiously, and are one of the most

Figure 11: Cross-table lateral technique

51

common orthopedic injuries seen in the emergency department (so yes, you should probably know this cold). These fractures can be considered intra-capsular, meaning that if displaced, they may result in disruption of the blood supply to the femoral head, risking *avascular necrosis of the femoral head*. They are described by location as either subcapital, transcervical, or basicervical. Refer to your atlas to better visualize these locations. Also note that basicervical fractures are managed differently as described below. Hip fractures can occur from high or low energy traumas, or also with cyclical loading as seen in athletes. The most common mechanism is a fall by an elderly person (with osteoporosis). Patients with displaced femoral neck fractures present with the extremity **shortened , abducted,** and **externally rotated.** With regards to radiographic evaluation, AP view of the pelvis, along with a cross-table lateral view of the proximal femur are sufficient. *A cross-table lateral view is obtained by flexing the uninjured hip and knee to 90 degrees and aiming the beam into the groin, perpendicular to the femoral neck* (Figure 11).

Femoral neck fractures can be classified using the **Garden classification:**

1. Valgus impacted
2. Complete, non-displaced fracture
3. Complete, partially displaced fracture
4. Complete, completely displaced

~Differentiating between Garden types 3 and 4 can be done by assessing the trabecular line patterns. In type 3, the lines will be perpendicular to the acetabulum as the displacement is incomplete, and type 4 will have trabecular lines parallel to the acetabulum.

Another important classification system to understand, although not as commonly used, is the **Pauwel classification.** This describes the fracture line by its angle compared to a horizontal line:

- Type 1: **< 30 degrees**
- Type 2: **30-70 degrees**
- Type 3: **> 70 degrees**

- The greater the angle, the more unstable the fracture due to an *increase in shear force.*

Unless the patient is at an extreme medical risk for surgery, operative treatment is the preferred management to restore hip function. Another incidence where operative management can be reconsidered is if the patient was non-ambulatory prior to the injury. But the caveat is that pain control itself may warrant fixation. In particular, if the patient is young, URGENT REDUCTION is essential. Minimally displaced fractures are pinned in situ with three cancellous screws (gold standard). These screws should be placed in an inverted triangle shape. Displaced fractures in the elderly population are treated with replacing the femoral head (termed hemiarthroplasty) or the entire joint (total hip arthroplasty). As a general rule (but of course each case is patient-specific), elderly patients with Types 1 or 2 fractures get ORIF with parallel screws, and Types 3 or 4 receive a hemiarthroplasty. Again, you must take into consideration the several factors relating to patient function and goals as mentioned earlier. One incidence where a total hip arthroplasty is strongly considered is when the patient has a history of *prior hip pain,* which indicates pre-existing osteoarthritis that may benefit from a total rather than a hemi.

Note: Early bed-to-chair mobilization is essential to avoid the risk of complications, including atelectasis, venous stasis, and pressure ulcers. Thus, you will see that patients are motivated to stand on their prosthesis as tolerated as soon as post-operative day 1 (considering their pain tolerance and pre-operative function). You will learn to appreciate that the advent of hip replacements is one of the more remarkable treatment options in our day. To have an individual walk again who was previously plagued by degenerative disease is an incredible skill of an orthopedist.

Important anatomy

- Normal femoral neck/shaft angle is *~120-135 degrees.*
- Understanding the positioning of the femoral head in the acetabulum is important to better comprehend normal ranges of motion as well as ideal alignment during hip replacement surgery:

- o   Acetabular anteversion is ~*10-15 degrees*
- o   Acetabular inclination is ~*45 degrees*
- The head and neck are primarily supplied by the medial femoral circumflex artery (off of the profunda femoris).
- The medial circumflex artery runs *posterior to the quadratus femoris* muscle. It can rarely be injured in a posterior approach to the hip.
  - o   Main branch is the lateral epiphyseal
  - o   2nd main branch is the piriformis branch off of the inferior gluteal artery
- The *lateral femoral cutaneous nerve* runs near the ASIS and is susceptible to injury/compression, as in an anterior approach to the thigh (causes *meralgia paresthetica* – numbness and dysesthesias on lateral aspect of the hip & thigh). This can result from patients who wear their pants too tight causing compression on the nerve.

Intertrochanteric hip fractures are extremely common hip fractures, but in contrast to femoral neck fractures they are considered *extracapsular*. They often result from a direct impact to the greater trochanteric area as may occur in a fall. These fractures occur in cancellous bone, which as described earlier has an abundant blood supply so nonunion and osteonecrosis are *not* major problems as they are in femoral neck fractures. The clinical evaluation is the same as that for femoral neck fractures, since these patients also present with a short and externally rotated extremity. They may also complain of pain with log rolling. Log rolling is a physical exam maneuver where the clinician passively internally and externally rolls the entire leg with the patient supine, trying to elicit pain at the hip joint. It is important to note that many intertrochanteric fracture patients may present with variable time after injury (i.e. if they fall and are unable to get up), so it is important to be aware of potential concomitant dehydration, nutritional depletion, and venous thromboembolic disease prior to admitting. It is not uncommon to hear a story of a patient being found on the floor >24 hours after falling. Hemodynamic stability must also be assessed because as much as 2 full units of blood can hemorrhage into the thigh. The radiographic evaluation is similar to that of a femoral neck fracture (AP & Cross-table lateral films), and an additional physician-assisted internal rotation view may help clarify the fracture pattern.

These fractures are classified based on their stability; the main factor in stability is derived from the status of the *posteromedial cortex (calcar femorale)*. For example, in stable fractures, the posteromedial cortex remains intact compared to unstable patterns. 2 other factors that determine stability are the presence of *subtrochanteric extension* of the fracture, or a *reverse obliquity* pattern (described below).

Similar to fractures around the femoral neck, surgical intervention is the preferred treatment to allow for early mobilization and full weight-bearing with ambulation; Early ORIF should be done with a sliding hip screw (gold standard) or a cephalomedullary nail, depending on the fracture pattern as well as physician preference. For example, a sliding hip screw is contraindicated in a reverse obliquity type intertrochanteric fracture.

Note: It is important to confirm proper positioning of the screw in the femoral head after placing a sliding hip screw. This is done by using both AP and lateral films, and measuring the *"tip-to-apex"* distance. This refers to the distance from the tip of the screw and the apex of the femoral head. The combined values on both views should be <25 mm. If it is >25 mm, then *screw cut out* may occur. The **Evans classification** is used to describe the stability and number of fragments. As mentioned earlier, the 3 important factors are calcar comminution, subtrochanteric extension, and reverse obliquity pattern.

~ *Reverse obliquity* intertrochanteric fractures have a fracture line that extends from the medial-proximal cortex to the distal-lateral cortex. These fractures are significant because they allow for medial displacement of the femur, making it inherently unstable. Therefore, these fractures are treated as subtrochanteric fractures utilizing a blade plate, or more commonly a cephalomedullary nail.

There are a couple of unusual fracture patterns seen around the intertrochanteric area. **Basicervical fractures** are located just proximal to the intertrochanteric line. Anatomically, it lies on the femoral neck, but because it is extracapsular it is treated as an intertrochanteric fracture. Because of the location, basicervical fractures are at a greater risk for osteonecrosis compared to the more distal intertrochanteric fractures. They are also associated with a rotational component during fixation.

Another injury that is associated with high-energy trauma that can be particularly life-threatening is a **fracture of the femoral shaft.** These constitute an orthopedic emergency. Although associated injuries are common (commonly an *ipsilateral femoral neck fracture*), an index of suspicion should be in place when a limb is short and deformed. This is why a full-length femur is generally warranted when a patient sustains a femoral neck fracture. Two important complications to be aware of include *fat embolism* and *susbstantial blood loss.* The thigh is a potential source of significant blood loss as mentioned earlier (up to **2** units!). Treatment may consist of placing traction as soon as possible, although this is often debated. Traction will restore the length, and in turn aid in tamponading the bleed. Traction will also relieve the pain, and partially immobilize the fracture. Neurovascular assessment is always essential as in any orthopedic injury, paying particular attention to distal pulses. Also, be aware of compartment syndrome.

Anatomy is important to understand in femoral shaft fractures as various muscles will cause specific deforming forces. For example, the gluteus medius and minimus muscles will displace the proximal fragment in abduction, and the iliopsoas will flex and rotate the proximal fragment. Know the muscle attachments and compartments of the thigh! The gold standard of treatment for such fractures is *intramedullary nailing*. When performed within 24 hours with early bed-to-chair mobilization, it has been shown to *decrease pulmonary complications, decrease thromboembolic events, and decrease the hospital length of stay.* Early mobilization is also particularly important due to **Wolff's law.** This states that the remodeling of the bone will adapt to the external loads under which it is placed. Some particular complications that may result from femoral shaft fractures include pudendal nerve injury, femoral vessel injury, compartment syndrome, and heterotopic ossification. **Heterotopic ossification** is not specific to femoral shaft injuries, but can occur with a vast number of orthopedic injuries. This is when bone tissue forms in abnormal places (outside of the skeleton). Although indomethacin has been used for prophylaxis, the treatment is generally surgical resection.

Important anatomic considerations
- The femur is the largest and strongest bone in the body
- There are 3 compartments of the thigh: anterior, posterior, adductor/medial; fasciotomy to release the anterior/posterior compartments should be done from the lateral aspect, whereas the adductor compartment should be managed via a medial approach.
- The borders of the *Adductor Canal* (*Hunter's Canal*) are the sartorius, vastus medialus, and adductor longus. It begins at the apex of the femoral triangle, and contains the femoral vessels. Be aware of the neurovascular structures when placing screws medially around the middle 1/3 of the femur, as with a distal locking screw. When placing a traction pin, it is recommended to proceed from medial to lateral to avoid these structures.

Although not the most common of fractures, **patellar fractures** are disabling injuries that can severely limit ambulatory capacity. The function of the patella is to increase the leverage of the quadriceps. Interestingly, direct trauma is not the most common mechanism for sustaining a patellar fracture. The most common way is by forcible quadriceps contraction while the knee is in a semi-flexed position, as when a person stumbles and tries to save the fall. In this situation the strength of the patella is exceeded by the quadriceps, and typically results in a transverse fracture pattern. Regardless, these fractures can be classified in several ways depending on the description/location of the injury: stellate, comminuted, transverse, vertical, polar, nondisplaced etc. Patients typically present with limited mobility, along with pain, swelling, and tenderness of the knee. **Note:** if the portions of the quadriceps tendons that attach directly onto tibia remain intact, then active extension may be preserved! (Or with preservation of part of the retinaculum). Surgical intervention is usually indicated when there is articular *displacement or gapping >2mm* or if there is a *loss of the extensor mechanism.*

Important anatomy

- Do not confuse patellar fractures with *bipartite patella* (unfused congenital corner of the patella). These generally are in a superolateral position. They can be differentiated by looking at the fracture line, determining if it is smooth vs. rough.
- The blood supply to the quadriceps tendon arises from the geniculate arteries (medial, lateral)
- The quadriceps tendon attaches to the superior aspect of the patella
- The patellar tendon/ligament continues from the patella to the tibial tuberosity.

Patellar dislocation is when the patella completely subluxates, most commonly laterally out of the trochlear groove (the normal anatomic groove through which the patella tracks on knee flexion and extension. The mechanism is generally from an externally rotated and planted tibia with the knee in some flexion. This occurs more

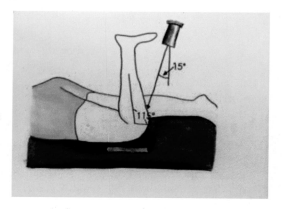

Figure 12: Sunrise view technique

commonly in women, most probably due to a greater generalized physiologic laxity in females. Patellar subluxation most commonly occurs due to weakness in the vastus medialis muscle. On physical exam patients may present with a hemarthrosis, an inability to flex the knee, or gross deformity. An apprehension test can be performed, where a positive test is indicated by the sensation of impending dislocation with a laterally directed force applied to the patella. This provocative maneuver is done with the knee in passive extension. In addition to the standard AP and lateral views, a *sunrise view* of both patellae should be obtained. *This view may be taken with the patient prone, knee flexed to about 115 degrees, and the beam at the patella about 15 degrees cephalad* (Figure 12).

Nonoperative management with casting or bracing is usually successful, with operative treatment being reserved for recurrent dislocations. **Note**: Simply straightening the knee may often lead to spontaneous relocation and reduction.

On radiographic evaluation, the lateral view x-ray of the knee depicts particular anatomic lines of importance:

> **Blumensaat's line** (Figure 13): This line projects from the roof of the intercondylar notch anteriorly, and should line up with the lower pole of the patella. This is assessed by a radiograph with the knee flexed at 30 degrees.

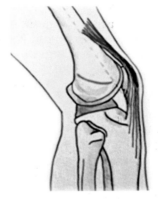

Figure 13: Blumensaat's line (red)

> **Insall-Salvati ratio:** This is the ratio of the length of the patellar ligament to the diagonal length of the patella should theoretically be 1.0 (normal). A ratio of 1.2 or higher indicates *patella alta*, and a ratio of 0.8 or below indicates *patella baja.* These terms refer to a high-riding patella and a low-riding patella, respectively. Patella baja may be seen if there is a complete quadriceps tendon rupture.

Important anatomy

- *Q-angle* is defined by a line drawn from the ASIS through the center of the patella, with a second line from the center of the patella to the tibial tubercle.
    - An increased Q angle predisposes one to dislocation/subluxation.
    - A normal Q angle ranges from 13 to 18 degrees, with females commonly having a greater angle
- Anatomic and mechanical axes are used to help determine lower extremity alignment

- Anatomic axis – line drawn along the axis of the femur
- Mechanical – line drawn between center of femoral head and intercondylar notch

Tibiofemoral dislocations (knee dislocations) are dangerous injuries due to the anatomically susceptible *popliteal artery.* Although rare, they are considered orthopedic emergencies. Due to the anatomy it is important to assess for vascular injury, and an *angiogram* may be indicated to look for tears in or around the popliteal artery. Knee dislocations require high-energy trauma to disrupt the multiple ligaments and soft tissue attachments that stabilize the knee. The extensive injury to the soft tissue oftentimes results in chronic knee instability. It is important to maintain a high index of suspicion as many may spontaneously reduce without intervention. **Note:** Assess *peroneal nerve function* due to its proximity to the knee joint. In management, most patients should probably be treated with ligament repair or reconstruction. Knee stiffness is one of the more common complications.

Important anatomy

- The gastrocnemius crosses the knee joint (2 heads), whereas the soleus does not. Keep this in mind when assessing which muscle is contributing to a plantar contracture of the foot. By flexing the knee, the gastrocnemius can be taken out of the equation.
- The iliotibial band extends from the tensor fascia lata, provides lateral support to the knee, and inserts on *Gerdy's tubercule.* This is a prominence just distal and lateral to the knee joint.
- The popliteus muscle provides resistance to external rotation. It inserts anterior and distal to the origin of the LCL. It's primary function is to disengage the "lock-in" mechanism of the femur on the tibia.

Tibial plateau fractures commonly occur secondary to trauma, with the mechanism being an axial load along with valgus or varus stresses. The plateau is the most proximal part of the tibia upon which the menisci sit. Therefore it is no surprise that many of these injuries have associated soft tissue damage and may have associated *meniscal tears* (medial/lateral corresponding to the side of fracture). **Note:** lateral fractures are more common than medial fractures. Understanding the Schatzker classification below will help depict the personalities of the different fracture patterns. On imaging such as CT scans, a way to differentiate the medial from the lateral tibia is that the medial aspect is more concave, looking almost like a golf tee (which is placed medial to the back leg, for those who play the sport). These fractures are classified based on the **Schatzker system:**

Type I: Split lateral plateau
Type II: Split lateral plateau, with depression (**MC**)
Type III: Lateral plateau with depression, NO split
Type IV: medial plateau fx (***consider angiogram***)
Type V: Bicondylar plateau fracture
Type VI: Plateau fracture with metadiaphyseal extension

Management depends on how displaced the fracture is. If there is a *< 3mm step off* or *< 5mm gapping*, it is considered non-displaced and a knee brace or cast with non-weight bearing status can be implemented for 6-8 weeks. If it is displaced, then ORIF is recommended with possible bone graft. CT is often very helpful to better determine the extent and personality of the lesion.

Important anatomy

- The medial plateau is *larger, concave* and *stronger,* so it is not as commonly fractured as the lateral. But when it is, always consider potential vascular injury.

As athletics have become a remarkable part of our society, more people are pushing the limits of their bodies, consequently risking greater injuries. With extensive throwing, jumping, diving, tackling, our sturdy frames become quite vulnerable. Very common injuries encountered during sports are those affecting the ligaments around the knees. These include the anterior cruciate (ACL), posterior cruciate (PCL), medial collateral (MCL), and lateral collateral (LCL) ligaments.

ACL injuries commonly occur with a twisting injury of a planted leg, often without any contact. The ACL functions to provide stability to the knee by preventing anterior translation of the tibia relative to the femur. It originates on the lateral aspect of the femur and inserts on the anterior aspect of the tibia between the intercondylar eminences (hence the name, anterior). A mnemonic for the insertions of the ACL and PCL you can use is "L-A-M-P." **L**ateral condyle – **A**CL – **M**edial condyle – **P**CL. The ACL consists of 2 bundles; the anteromedial, which is tight in flexion, and posterolateral, which is tight in extension. The blood supply is from the middle geniculate artery. The innervation is by the posterior articular nerve (off of the tibial nerve). The strength of the ACL can resist up to 2200 N of force. A lateral meniscal tear is generally associated with an acute ACL injury, whereas a medial meniscal tear is associated with a chronic ACL injury. The size of the ACL measures about 33mm x 11mm. These patients may describe a sensation of a "pop", accompanied by swelling and pain deep in the knee. Swelling tends to happen *rapidly* (compared to meniscal injuries) due to the development of a hemarthrosis. Remember that ligaments have a greater vascular supply than menisci, which depend more on diffusion for nutrients. The patient's gait may be indicative of an ACL injury as he or she may not actively extend the knee during ambulation (avoiding the use of the quadriceps muscle).

Although radiographs are generally not diagnostic, a pathognomonic finding for ACL tears is an avulsion fracture of the lateral tibial condyle, called a *Segond fracture.* The most sensitive physical maneuver is the Lachman's test. This is performed with the patient supine, and flexing the knee about 15 degrees. One hand grasps the distal femur and the other hand grasps the proximal tibia, and the examiner provides an anterior translation, assessing for a soft (abnormal) or firm endpoint. A firm endpoint is normal, whereas a soft endpoint indicates an inefficient ACL. The Lachman's test has a greater sensitivity than the anterior drawer test because when the knee is flexed to 90 degrees (as in the anterior drawer test), other soft tissue structures are stabilizing the knee giving a potential false negative. The most specific test is the Pivot shift test. This test takes advantage of the fact that the iliotibial (IT) band is an extensor in extension, and a flexor in flexion. As a valgus stress is placed on the extended knee, the tibia is internally rotated by the examiner to maximize the instability of the knee. As the knee is flexed, the IT band acts as a flexor and reduces the anterolateral subluxation back into places, causing a "clunk." This is better understood by watching an examiner perform this. ACL injuries are commonly associated with other injuries, termed the *terrible triad (ACL, MCL, and meniscal injury)*. For elderly, low-demand patients, physical therapy and lifestyle modifications may be the management of choice. For younger, more active patients, ACL reconstruction is a probable option with pre-operative bracing and physical therapy to strengthen the quadriceps and hamstrings.

In regards to ACL reconstruction, several different grafts may be used. The surgeon must create a femoral and a tibial tunnel into which the bony part of the graft will be placed. The femoral tunnel placement should be carried out with a 1-2 mm rim of bone between the tunnel and the posterior cortex of the femur. Anterior misplacement results in a knee that is tight in flexion and loose in extension. A posterior misplacement results in a knee that is the opposite. Although various grafts can be used, an autograft (patient's own tissue) is preferred due to efficiency and a lower chance of immune reaction. An example is a bone-patella-bone (BPB) graft using the patellar tendon. The maximal potential load until failure occurs is around 2600 N, which is a pretty impressive force when you think about it. A hamstring autograft can also be utilized, and the maximum load to failure is ~ 4000N. A hamstring graft makes use of a portion of the semitendinosis tendon. Although not used as commonly, a contralateral quadriceps tendon may also be an option.

The function of the PCL is to restrain posterior tibial translation/hyperflexion of the knee. It originates at the posterior tibia and inserts on the medial femoral condyle (remember "LAMP"). It's size measures around 38mm x 13mm. It also consists of 2 bands, one being anterolateral (which is tight in flexion), and one that is posteromedial (which is tight in extension). The blood supply is from the middle geniculate artery, just like the ACL's vascular supply. During arthroscopy, there are meniscofemoral ligaments that may be mistaken for the PCL. These include the ligaments of Humphrey (anterior to PCL) and Wrisberg (posterior to PCL); they run from the posterior horn of the lateral meniscus to the lateral aspect of the medial femoral condyle. Refer to an atlas to better visualize these structures to make it easier to recognize on an arthroscopic evaluation.

PCL injuries occur secondary to hyperxtension of the knee, or an excessive anterior to posterior force on the tibia (as a dashboard injury in a motor vehicle collision). Although the patient may present similarly with a swollen knee, the *posterior drawer test* is the maneuver that will help identify a PCL injury. This is done by applying a posterior force to the proximal tibia, with the knee flexed to 90 degrees, and assessing the translation for a soft (abnormal) or firm (normal) endpoint. Based on the displacement, PCL injuries are graded I-III. The *quadriceps active test* can also be utilized where the patient tries to extend the knee flexed at 90 degrees, and you observe for anterior translation of the tibia. Although MRI is the most accurate test for all of these ligamentous injuries, a lateral stress view may possibly be useful in the diagnosis of a PCL injury.

Medial and Lateral collateral ligament injuries occur due to excess valgus and varus forces, respectively. They may present with joint instability and tenderness. The MCL is the most commonly injured ligament of the knee. There are 2 layers, and they consist of the superficial and deep medial collateral ligaments.

Meniscal injuries are one of the most common reasons for knee surgery (medial more common than lateral). The tears can occur in various patterns, such as longitudinal, horizontal, bucket handle, parrot beak, and radial (use google image to better visualize). Radiographically, a bucket handle lesion may present as a "double PCL sign" on MRI. The best way you will learn this is by repetition and continuing to read MRIs (it is not easy). These injuries generally occur during a distinctly recalled acute knee injuries, oftentimes associated with a popping sensation (similar to ACL). For example, athletes may come in describing a distinct twisting motion of a planted leg that caused a "pop" in the knee. In contrast to ligament tears, knee swelling tends to be *gradual.* Patients may complain of "locking" and "clicking" with certain movements after the inciting event. Physical exam is particularly helpful for suspected injuries, with *joint line tenderness* being an important clue. The *McMurray test* is a provocative test that is used; it is done by flexing the knee, providing a varus or valgus stress at the knee, and bringing the knee back into extension. A positive test is indicated by a palpable "click" with a possible reproduction of pain.

The anatomy of these cartilaginous structures is important as different locations of the lesions are managed differently. The peripheral aspect of the meniscus is vascular, and is broken down into 3 zones. Injury to this area can be treated by possibly fixing the tear. In contrast, the more central lesions must be debrided as they have a poor ability to heal due to the deficient blood supply. A meniscectomy is often performed for central lesions to reduce the pain and to reduce the possibility of early onset osteoarthritis; the frayed parts of the meniscus can constantly rub and irritate the bone. The **Fairbanks** system was derived to describe post-meniscectomy degenerative joint changes as visualized on radiograph. They include *squaring of the condyles, peaking of the eminences, ridging,* and *joint space narrowing.*

Ankle sprains are one of the most common reasons for ED visits (and so you should understand them rather comprehensively). On a basic level, one common mechanism of injury is from inversion of the ankle and tearing of the lateral ligaments, usually the anterior talofibular ligament (mnemonic: **ATF - A**lways **T**orn **F**irst). The 2nd most commonly torn ligament that resists inversion is the *calcaneofibular ligament.* The 3rd ligament to tear if the sprain were even worse would be the strongest of the lateral ligaments, the posterior talofibular ligament (Grade III). These injuries tend to heal well, but repeated sprains as seen in athletes and dancers can result in chronic ankle instability. The diagnosis is essentially based off of the history, but of course MRI can visualize the soft tissue if needed. There is usually pain after a twisting injury to the ankle. For example, a basketball player comes down for a rebound and lands on another player's foot, resulting in excess inversion and a resulting tear in ligaments. **Note:** eversion injuries of the same caliber tend to cause *fractures* due to the toughness of the deltoid ligament. Depending on the grade of the common sprain, swelling and tenderness is usually present distal and anterior to the lateral malleolus (corresponding to the anatomical location of the ligaments).

As this is such a common injury, judicious imaging is of particular importance. This can be determined using the *Ottawa rules* for ankle fractures. This essentially states that imaging of the ankle is indicated if there is an inability to bear weight immediately after the injury, with tenderness over the posterior aspect of the medial malleolus or the lateral malleolus, or tenderness over the base of the navicular or base of the 5th metatarsal. On imaging, x-rays can be normal or may show small bits of avulsed bone from the tip of the lateral malleolus. **Note:** as most orthopedic injuries call for 2 views 90 degrees to each other, *ankle injuries should get a third view called the Mortise view; this is with the ankle in 15 degrees of internal rotation.* The mortise is defined by the plafond (distal tibial articular surface), and lateral and medial malleoli. The reason for this view is to better visualize the medial joint space. Depending on the extent of injury, rest/ice/elevation/compression (RICE) and NSAIDS may be the treatments of choice. An ankle brace for several weeks may be of benefit to prevent re-injury to the unstable ankle. If pain persists for greater than around 8 weeks after conservative treatment then an MRI is indicated. Seldom indicated, but completely torn ligaments with continued pain and injury may be candidates for anatomic reconstruction and tenodesis.

Anatomical consideration: The normal ranges of motion of the ankle are about 30 degrees of dorsiflexion and about 45 degrees of plantar flexion.

Ankle fractures can occur with excessive forces on the ankle while the ankle is in particular positions. It is extremely important to thoroughly understand these mechanisms and the associated fractures, as you are undoubtedly going to see them. That is a promise. These are briefly described by the Lauge-Hansen classification below, but do read up on the mechanisms and phases in detail. For example, understand the sequence of events occurring in "Supination External Rotation" mechanisms, which ligaments tear in which order, and the presence of an associated specific spiral fracture pattern of the distal fibula (which runs from anteroinferior to posterosuperior).

The **Lauge-Hansen classification** organizes ankle fractures by injury sequences; it takes into account the position of the foot at time of injury, and the direction of the deforming force. These can be remembered by the menomic "SAD-SER-PR":

- **S**upination-**Ad**duction (a/w Weber A) ; a unique feature of this is a depiction of a *vertical fracture of the medial malleolus*
- **S**upination- **e**xternal **r**otation (a/w Weber B); Note: This is the most common mechanism of injury. It is important to understand the sequence of injury also. In short, there is injury to the anterior inferior tibiofibular ligament (AITFL) → lateral malleolus fx (spiral fx is usually anteroinferior to posterosuperior) → posterior tibiofibular injury (PITFL) → medial malleolus fx
- **Pr**onation-abduction (a/w Weber C)
- **Pr**onation-external rotation

Management of these patients has to do with the stability of the injury. All dislocations should be reduced immediately (to decrease post injury swelling and limit neurovascular damage). When they present in the ED, the leg will generally be placed in a splint with two components (a posterior slab, and a stir-up). These will be better understood when you watch and do your first splint. It is very important to understand this as you can be of significant help to the resident physician who will be managing this injury. When possible, it may be in your best interest to gather the supplies, measure out the components of the splint, and have everything ready and available by the time the doctor is ready. This goes for any procedure in which time can be saved. Trust me, they will appreciate it.

When 1 malleolus is involved, the fracture is usually considered stable. If both malleoli are involved, or a "bimalleolar equivalent" is considered, then the injury is deemed unstable; bimalleolar fractures are intra-articular in nature. A bimalleolar equivalent is when there is no obvious medial malleolus fracture, but when stressing the joint by external rotation, there is an increased gap in the medial joint space. A stable, non-displaced injury can be treated with a short leg cast. An unstable, displaced fracture requires ORIF and possible syndesmosis fixation. Lateral malleolar fractures may be managed using a lag screw (described under "Screws") or wires. Medial malleolar fracture management is controversial; many physicians advocate no treatment, but in general, it should be operated on if there is concomitant syndesmotic injury or a persistently wide joint space after fibular reduction. **When the deltoid ligament at the medial ankle is injured, the talus most commonly shifts laterally in the plafond.**

On radiographic evaluation, there are specific measurements that should be considered to determine the stability of the different parts of the ankle. This is best learned by practicing reading and

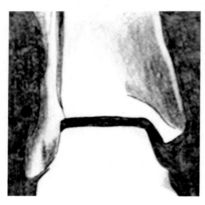

Figure 14: Medial clear space

interpreting these x-rays. The joint space around the plafond should be even all around. If there is incongruency then there is possible medial or lateral disruption of the ankle ligaments. If there is an isolated fibular fracture it is important to remember to check for medial disruption. **The most important way to assess the competency of the deltoid ligament is by an** *external rotation stress radiograph;* stress radiographs are useful in determining the amount of ligamentous laxity present following trauma. **A medial clear space of > 5mm** with external rotation stress applied to a dorsiflexed ankle is predictive of deltoid disruption and/or a lateral talar shift (Figure 14). This test is done by dorsiflexing the ankle, internally rotating the tibia, and externally rotating the ankle. A positive stress view may indicate syndesmotic injury, and is oftentimes considered a "bimalleolar equivalent." The syndesmosis is the ligamentous structures which give the higher ankle stability. It consists of the AITFL, PITFL, interosseus ligament, and transverse tibiofibular ligament (TTFL). Intraoperatively, the *cotton test* is used to stress the joint; this is done by pulling the fibula laterally and observing for any widening of the syndesmosis. On an AP film, you should also assess the **tibiofibular overlap** (should be at least 10 mm), and **the tibial clear space** (should be <5 mm). Abornmalities of these measurements also may indicate damage to the syndesmosis.

Ankle fractures can also be classified according to the level of their associated fibular fractures; a known classification system is the **Danis-Weber system.** It is important to note that *the more proximal the injury, the greater the risk of injury to the syndesmosis and the greater the instability.* The Danis-Weber classification breaks down such ankle fractures into 3 types (A, B, and C):

> **A:** fibular fracture *distal to plafond*
> **B:** fibular fracture *at the plafond*; Weber B fractures generally warrant a stress radiograph (remember, >5mm space indicates a "bimalleolar equivalent" injury, which is inherently unstable)
> **C:** fibular fracture *proximal to the plafond* (almost always associated with syndesmotic fracture)

Important Anatomy

- The structures passing posterior to the medial malleolus are important to understand, especially during ORIF procedures. They can be remembered using the mnemonic *Tom Dick And Nervous Harry*; **T** = tibialis posterior; **D** = Flexor digitorum longus; **A** = posterior tibial artery; **N** = tibial nerve; **H** = Flexor Hallucis Longus
- The common peroneal nerve runs about 12 cm proximal to the lateral malleolus

The **plafond /pilon** itself can be fractured and is generally the result of high-energy mechanisms (commonly axial compression). A plafond means "ceiling," and in this context refers to end of the tibia that involves the articulating surface (looks sort of like a ceiling to the ankle joint on an AP view). These fractures present with intense swelling and pain, and may require full trauma evaluations and serial neurovascular exams. The swelling complicates early open treatment, which may substantiate delayed surgical intervention for several days. There may also be evidence of an open fracture as this part of the tibia is relatively close to the skin. These fractures can be classified by the **Ruedi and Allgower classification system**, which is based on the comminution and displacement of the articular surface:

1. Nondisplaced
2. Displaced with minimal articular comminution
3. Significant comminution

Nondisplaced fractures can be treated with a long leg cast for six weeks, whereas ORIF is indicated for most displaced injuries. Again, ORIF may be delayed to allow for the swelling to decrease. Maintaining fibular length and stabilizing the articular joint are both important goals for operative fixation. There are 3 commonly seen fragments that are seen with pilon fractures: a medial fragment, a Chaput fragment (anterolateral), and a Volkmann fragment (posterolateral).

A **Maisonneuve fracture** is an ankle injury with a fracture of the *proximal fibula, along with a complete syndesmotic disruption*; it is a pronation-external rotation type injury. The force is understood to transmit distally from the ankle through the interosseus membrane to the proximal fibula. There will be proximal fibula tenderness, which should give you suspicion as these fractures may be missed on radiographs; they may also need stress views to better visualize the instability.

As you may have noticed, eponyms are a common way to define and describe orthopedic lesions. Of importance with ankle fractures are the following. An avulsion fracture of the distal tibia by the AITFL is termed a **Tillaux fracture.** The counterpart to this lesion on the fibula is termed the **LeForte-Wagstaffe** fracture. An avulsion fracture of the posterior malleolus is termed a **curbstone fx.**

Important anatomy

- The syndesmosis is an organization of ligaments providing primary support of the ankle (AITFL, PITFL, TTFL, interosseus membrane). A tear will cause the fibula to displace laterally
- The deltoid ligament at the medial ankle is the primary restraint to eversion and external rotation of the ankle.
- 2 important attachments to the fibular head
  - lateral collateral ligament

- biceps femoris

Another important fracture about the ankle is that of the **talar neck**. The mechanism of this injury is commonly from a high-energy forced dorsiflexion. The *posterior tibial artery* (major blood supply for talus via <u>retrograde</u> vessels) is in vicinity during such injuries, and so a displaced talar neck fracture may result in osteonecrosis of the body of the talus with poor outcome. The Canal and Sinus branches are particularly important. Displaced neck fractures actually constitute an orthopedic emergency. For optimal view of the talar neck, a *Canale view* should be utilized. The positioning is in maximum equinus, 15 degrees eversion, and the x-ray beam about 75 degrees cephalad from horizontal. A *Broden view* can also be utilized. This is with the leg internally rotated about 45 degrees, and films taken at 10, 20, 30, and 40 degrees of cephalic tilt. This will help to particularly visualize the posterior facet of the calcaneus. A <u>positive</u> prognostic factor that indicates a lesser risk of AVN is the presence of resorption of subchondral bone on the x-ray. This is seen as a *lucency*, and indicates *fracture healing.* This is termed the **Hawkins sign.** All cases require an emergent closed reduction. A short leg cast can be used for 8-12 weeks, or for displaced fractures, urgent ORIF to decreases the risk of AVN. In addition to AVN, *varus malunion* is a potential complication of this injury, as is *subtalar arthritis.* A fracture of the lateral process of the talus is commonly called a *snowboarder's fracture,* which does not pose as great of a risk of AVN as does a fracture to the neck.

Talar neck fractures may be classified using the **Hawkins Classification**, which helps to *predict the risk of AVN*:

> Type I: Nondisplaced (*tx = percutaneous pin)*
> Type II: Associated subtalar subluxation or dislocation
> Type III: Associated subtalar AND tibiotalar dislocation
> Type IV: Subtalar dislocation, tibiotalar dislocation, AND associated talonavicular dislocation.
>
> > *Types 1-4 have risks of AVN at around 10%, 40%, 90%, and 100% respectively.*

71

Calcaneal fractures occur from traumatic axial loading. For this reason, about 10% of these are associated with *vertebral injuries* (order a lumbar films!). The calcaneal pain may be so significant that the patient is unaware of the spine injury, so it is important to *carefully examine the spine*. Neurovascular examination should consist of assessing for compartment syndrome of the foot, which may result in a clawing of the toes (know that there are 9 main compartments that make up the foot). The majority of these fractures are *intra-articular* in nature. This is important as intra-articular fractures affect the subtalar joint, especially the posterior facet. It is crucial to understand the anatomical landmarks of the calcaneus, such as the superior articular surface. It consists of the posterior facet, which is the largest of the facets and constitutes the majority of the weight-bearing area. The prognosis is rather remarkable with an approximate 40% complication rate, including post-traumatic subtalar osteoarthritis and long-term disability.

Radiologic assessment requires AP, lateral, and *oblique foot* views. A *Harris view* will help better visualize these injuries. This is taken by dorsiflexing the foot with the beam 45 degrees cephalad to the heel. CT scan is the gold standard in defining the fracture personality. Lateral radiographs may show particular lines and angles that can aid in evaluation.

Boehler's angle (Figure 15) – a line is drawn from the highest point of the anterior calcaneus to the highest point of the posterior facet. A tangential line is drawn from the posterior facet to the superior edge of the

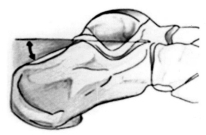

Figure 15: Boehler's angle

posterior tuberosity (insertion of the Achilles' tendon). The normal angle is between 20 and 40 degrees. A decrease in this angle indicates that the weight-bearing posterior facet has collapsed, causing the body weight to shift anteriorly. Subtalar incongruity may also be indicated by a double density on radiograph.

72

- *Gissane (crucial) angle* (Figure 16) – These angles are between 130 and 145 degrees and are visualized beneath the lateral process of the talus. An increase in this angle indicates a collapse of the posterior facet.

Calcaneal fractures are classified as intra- or extra-articular. An example of an extra-articular fracture includes an avulsion of the posterior tuberosity (by the Achilles), which is common in diabetics and osteoporotics. Note: In the pediatric population, the calcaneal tuberosity may develop an apophysitis (inflammation of the bony protuberance) that is termed **Sever's disease.**

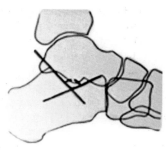

Figure 10: Critical angle of Gissane

As CT scans are commonly used to better delineate these fractures, a radiographic classification system is used based on the CT scan findings called the **Sanders Classification.** This is based on the number and location of articular fragments on the coronal images. This is organized into 4 types, as per particular fracture lines.

Treatment can be either cast immobilization (for nondisplaced), closed reduction with percutaneous pinning, or ORIF. Wound complications are not uncommon, and are particularly greater in smokers and diabetics (as is the case with most injuries). For a patient with a comminuted fracture who is a younger working person, *primary subtalar fusion* is a possible indication.

Plantar Fasciitis is one of the most commonly encountered orthopedic conditions seen in the clinic. This refers to microtears in the origin of the plantar fascia (the connective tissue that supports the arch of the foot), usually at the origin on the calcaneus. The cause is from repetitive trauma and chronic overuse, common in dancers and runners. Patients will complain of sharp heel pain, classically worse when first getting out of bed, relieved by ambulation, and worse after prolonged standing. On exam, one will note tenderness at the medial calcaneal tuberosity. Although radiographs are generally negative, heel spurs may be present. The management of these patients is usually non-operative, combining analgesics with lifestyle modifications. This includes stretching, night splints, and heel inserts for the shoe.

Lisfranc injury (tarsometatarsal fracture-dislocation) is a condition characterized by disruption between the *medial cuneiform* and the *base of the 2nd metatarsal.* This can be a fracture or simply ligamentous injury. The mechanism of this injury occurs most commonly from forced plantar flexion of the forefoot, so be sure to keep in mind of other possible tarsal fractures. Forced plantar flexion can occur from any of motor accidents, sports injuries, or falls, so it is important to keep on your differential list. The inexperienced eye commonly misses this diagnosis as radiograph findings are subtle, but its identification is crucial due to its prognosis. (Weight bearing views may be necessary to observe displacement). In regards to x-rays, a *>2mm* space between the 2nd metatarsal base and cuneiform is pathologic. This is an indication for surgical fixation. A *fleck sign* may also be noticed on radiograph, which is a small bony fragment in the space, indicating an avulsion of the Lisfranc ligament.

Lisfranc injuries can result in progressive foot deformity, chronic pain and dysfunction. On exam, there may be mid-foot swelling, some plantar bruising, and tenderness. An instability test may be performed to test for dorsal subluxation of the joint. Nonoperative management via cast immobilization for 8 weeks may be indicated for certain candidates i.e. nondisplaced fractures. Operative intervention (indicated if >2mm widening) include ORIF, external fixation, and closed reduction with percutaneous pinning. An altered gait pattern or limp may be a resulting complication of these injuries.

Important anatomy:

- The Lisfranc ligament is essential in stabilizing the second metatarsal as well as maintaining the arch of the midfoot
- This ligament tightens with pronation & abduction of the forefoot

74

Other fractures involving the midfoot area are those of the metatarsals, the proximal 5th metatarsal in particular (the "base" of the metatarsal). The proximal 5th metatarsal is further divided into 3 zones, numbered from proximal to distal. An avulsion fracture off of the tuberosity (Zone 1) is caused by the *lateral band of the plantar aponeurosis* or the *peroneus brevis* muscle tendons. The proximal 5th metatarsal fracture of Zone 2 is called the **Jones fracture,** which is anatomically defined as the metadiaphyseal junction. This area is a <u>watershed zone</u>, making it particularly susceptible to nonunion if there is injury to the nutrient artery. Fractures to Zone 3, referred to as "dancer's fractures," are not at a great risk of vascular compromise. Metatarsal fractures can also be stress fractures as seen in runners. A Zone 1 fracture can be managed with a hard shoe. Injuries to Zones 2 and 3 can be managed with a short leg non-weight bearing cast. ORIF may be necessary for certain candidates, such as athletes.

Achilles rupture and tendonitis-

Achilles tendon ruptures are usually from overuse injuries, or a sudden increase in use in a deconditioned individual. The Achilles tendon is the largest tendon in the body and consists of the gastrocnemius and soleus tendons. The attachment is to the posterior tuberosity of the calcaneus (where a deformity or tenderness may be appreciated). Patients may complain of a loud "pop" sound, as well as a sharp pain described as "being kicked in the leg." The rupture occurs about 3cm above the insertion of the tendon due to the fact that it is a watershed area. The **Thompson test** is generally positive (squeezing the superficial posterior compartment of the calf does not cause the normal plantar flexion as should by simulating calf contraction). **Note:** False negatives may occur if accessory ankle flexors are squeezed together with the contents of the superficial posterior leg compartment. Deformity may also be noted on physical exam as a space from a retracted tendon. Either conservative or operative management can be used to restore the strength and function of the gastrocnemius-soleus complex. Conservative treatment begins *with immobilization of the foot in equinus* position (plantar flexion), with progressive weight-bearing,

> Accessory ankle flexors include the posterior tibialis, flexor digitorum longus, flexor halluces longus, or accessory soleus muscles

exercises, and heel lifts, transitioning back to normal shoes. Surgical treatment is often preferred for younger and more athletic patients, and may decrease the risk of re-rupture.

Pediatric Orthopedics

As children are poor historians, it is important for the clinician to use keen diagnostic skills in assessing a pediatric orthopedic case. Generally speaking, there are a few characteristics of pediatric bone that you should take into consideration when deciding management. Firstly, fractures in children tend to heal more quickly than in adults. This can be attributed to the increase in levels of growth hormone (a known potent stimulator for fracture healing). Additionally, pediatric bone has a thicker and stronger periosteum, so complete fractures through both cortices is uncommon. An additional characteristic unlike that in adults is that children have considerable remodeling potential, allowing for substantial fracture deformity and angulation tolerances. This is depicted well in the management of clavicle fractures in pediatrics. A fracture can be completely displaced and shortened to some extent, and if the physician decides to treat it non-operatively there is a great chance that the bone will heal back to its normal alignment. The bone metabolism is such that the breakdown and build up of bone and callus over a span of time will remodel the injured area back to a normal position. This is of course only until a certain age and depends on maturity.

Despite these features, children are particularly predisposed to injuries since they are active by nature. An especially vulnerable location of bone injuries in this population is the physis (growth plate), which is weaker than the surrounding bone to external forces. In addition, ligaments in children are functionally stronger than bone; therefore injuries that produce sprains in adults may result in fractures in children. Adding to the skeletal immaturity, the vascular development not being complete heightens the risk of osteonecrosis/avascular necrosis.

Of particular importance in the pediatric population are the injuries that involve the physes as these can cause issues with growth. These are classified as **Salter-Harris fractures**, and are grouped according to the extent of the injury ranging from Type I to Type V (Figure 20). Treatment also varies accordingly. For example, if the growth plate is in one piece and the displacement is lateral as in a type 1, then closed reduction may provide adequate management. If the fracture crosses the epiphyses or growth plate and involves the joint, then precise alignment with open reduction internal fixation (ORIF) is required to prevent complete growth arrest or limb length inequalities.

When Salter-Harris type III fractures involve the *anterolateral distal tibial epiphysis*, this is called a **juvenile tillaux fracture.** These fractures are

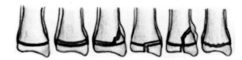

most commonly seen in the early *teenage* years, and are caused by

Figure 11: Salter-Harris classification, normal and Types 1-5

external rotation forces causing *the anterior inferior tibiofibular ligament* (AITFL) to avulse the fragment. Such avulsion fractures do not occur as commonly in adults because the ligament tends to give out instead of avulsing the bone. The avulsed piece of metaphyseal bone that is carried with the epiphysis is termed the *Thurston Holland fragment.*

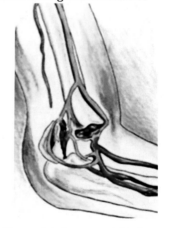

Another commonly encountered fracture resulting from bending forces that *incompletely* fracture the bone are called **greenstick fractures**

The natural instinct to break a fall with outstretched hands poses risk to numerous musculoskeletal injuries. Particularly of note in children (considering a child's joint can hyperextend more than an adult's), are **supracondylar fractures**

Figure 18: Supracondylar fx

of the humerus. This is represented by a break of the distal humerus with the fracture commonly opening *anteriorly*. This is an essential diagnosis to make as vascular (*brachial artery*) and nerve (*anterior interosseus)* injuries can easily occur and result in a subsequent *Volkmann contracture* (described below). When the elbow is splinted in substantial flexion as recommended, the *brachial artery* can become squeezed in the fracture site and spasm off! This results in ischemic necrosis and subsequent scarring of the forearm musculature, which was previously mentioned as a "Volkmann's contracture (Figure 19)." Although these fractures infrequently need surgery, it is important to vigilantly monitor for the development of compartment syndrome and/or neurovascular compromise. These fractures also tend to heal with a varus or valgus deformity (more commonly varus), and it is recommended to treat with closed reduction and pinning (Types II and III). Be aware of the proximity of the ulnar nerve if considering a medial approach with pinning as it courses medially along the distal arm. Imaging should assess the *anterior humeral line* to demonstrate normal or abnormal elbow alignment. This is a line drawn the surface of the humerus on a lateral film and should intersect the middle third of the capitellum. A displaced supracondylar fracture would demonstrate this line being anterior to the capitellum. The *radiocapitellar line* is also used on radiograph to determine elbow alignment. This line is drawn from the neck of the radial head and should intersect the capitellum. If it does not, then a radial head dislocation can be considered.

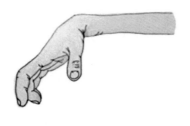

Figure 19: Volkmann's contracture

It is important to know the pattern of ossification of the bones around the elbow. They are commonly remembered by the mnemonic "Come Rub My Tree of Love" – Capitellum, Radial head, Medial epicondyle, Trochlea, Olecranon, Lateral epicondyle." The chronological age of the patient corresponding to the pattern is 1-3-5-7-9-11. (Some authors suggest that those numbers correspond to a female's development, and 2-4-6-8-10-12 are for a male). Also note that this is the order of ossification, and when it comes to fusion, the last bone to fuse is the medial epicondyle.

These fractures can be classified according to the **Gartland classification:**

Type I: Nondisplaced
Type II: Displaced with an intact posterior cortex
Type III: Completely displaced

Another fracture of the pediatric elbow is that of the **lateral condylar physis.** These often have less promising results in comparison to supracondylar fractures. These fractures disrupt the connection with the proximal radius (displaced laterally) due to the loss of stability from the distal humerus. This must be differentiated from a fracture of the entire distal humeral physis, in which the proximal radius is intact. Nondisplaced fractures can be treated with immobilization of the forearm in neutral with the elbow flexed to 90 degrees. If a treatment is delayed for several weeks, *closed treatment* is recommended regardless of the degree of displacement. This is due to the increased risk of *osteonecrosis* with late open reduction.

The mnemonic "SALTER" can be used to help remember the first five types. This mnemonic requires the reader to imagine the bones as long bones, with the epiphyses at the base.

- I – S = **Slip**. Fracture of the *cartilage* of the physis
- II – A = **Above**. The fracture lies Above the physis, or **A**way (proximal) from the joint
- III – L = **Lower**. The fracture is below the physis in the epiphysis (distal)
- IV – TE = **Through Everything**. The fracture is through the metaphysis, physis, and epiphysis
- V – R = **Rammed (crushed)**. The physis has been crushed.

Child Abuse

An unfortunate truth in our society is that child abuse is fairly prevalent (>1%). It is important to maintain a high index of suspicion and obtain a radiographic skeletal survey if abuse is suspected. Child protective services should be notified immediately, and the patient should be admitted. There are several characteristics of injuries that should raise suspicion for child abuse:

Transverse femur fracture or humeral fracture in young child	History inconsistent with fracture pattern
Fractures in various stages of healing	Inconsistent history on repeating story
Bruises in areas not overlying bony prominences	History not consistent with developmental milestones
Rib fractures	Skull fractures
Delay in seeking care	

Common pediatric conditions

Scoliosis is a term that is heard quite early as it is commonly diagnosed on school screening exams. More common in girls, this condition refers to an abnormal curvature of the spine, particularly a lateral bending with a rotational component. The etiology of this disorder can stem from various issues including congenital (abnormal vertebra), neuromuscular disease (muscle imbalance), and idiopathic (most common). Pain is usually not an issue. On the "Adam's forward bending test," there may be spinal deformities resulting in a classic rib "hump." A full spine x-ray is taken and the Cobb technique is utilized to determine the angle of the curve, which aids in determining management. The Cobb angle is measured by using the most superior and inferior parts of the curve, drawing parallel lines from vertebral endplates, and measuring the angle formed by the two intersecting parallel lines. In regard to treatment, patients with an angle of < 25 degrees are generally managed conservatively with exercises, stretches, and observation. For those with angles between 25 and 40 degrees, bracing is an effective option for halting the progression during a child's growth phase. Patients with large curves (> 40 degrees) are generally treated surgically by spinal fusion to partially correct the curve in attempt to minimize the associated cardiac and respiratory compromise. These are of course not definite numbers as different clinicians may use different scales.

Hematogenous osteomyelitis is not uncommon in the pediatric population due to the metaphysis being highly vascular with a fairly sluggish blood flow. On exam, children will refuse to use the affected extremity and may complain of localized pain. Erythema, warmth, swelling, and tenderness is also appreciated, often accompanied by fever, leukocytosis, and an increased ESR (>40). X-rays should be obtained, but *may initially be normal* as osteolytic changes take several days to develop. A positive x-ray of osteomyelitis is indicated with the presence of soft tissue swelling and periosteal elevation. *The most sensitive and specific test is MRI with gadolinium.* Blood cultures should be obtained, but it is important to note that cultures are positive less than 60% of the time. *The most common offending organism is Staphylococcus aureus.* **Note:** Children with sickle cell have an increased incidence of *Salmonella* infection. Nonetheless, *S. Aureus* is still the most common organism causing osteomyelitis. Management is usually nonoperative with IV antibiotics for 6 weeks, UNLESS an abscess or necrotic, sequestered bone is present, in which case surgical debridement may be indicated.

The **Kocher criteria** is used for suspected pediatric septic arthritis of the hip (to differentiate from transient synovitis) and includes the following factors:
- Non-weight bearing
- ESR >40
- Fever
- WBC > 12,000

Developmental dysplasia of the hip is a condition where the femoral head is not deeply seated in the acetabulum, making it vulnerable to complete dislocation. The diagnosis is usually made clinically at birth by assessing the stability of the hip; this is done using the Ortolani and Barlow's maneuvers. *Barlow's* is performed by adducting and depressing the femur posteriorly to potentially dislocate a susceptible hip. ("B" for pushing BACK). *Ortolani's* test reduces a dislocated hip with anterior elevation and abduction of the femur (Figure 21). The dislocation commonly occurs superiorly and anteriorly. It is important to note that both of these tests become

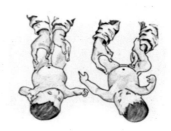

Figure 21: Barlow (left) & Ortolani (right)

negative after 3 months as soft tissue contractures develop. Additionally on exam, the condition may present *with uneven gluteal folds*. *Ultrasound* is a highly sensitive test; X-rays are not ideal considering the hip is not yet calcified. **Note:** bilateral cases are often missed due to both hips seeming similar on exam and x-ray. The goal of treatment is to maintain a concentric reduction, particularly to prevent the later development of osteoarthritis. Treatment consists of bracing using a Pavlik harness (Figure 22) for 2 weeks (then reassessing). Children diagnosed older than 6 months generally require surgical correction.

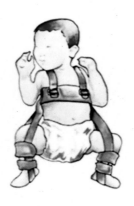

Figure 22: Pavlik harness

Note: Hip pathology in the pediatric population may present solely as referred *knee pain.*

Legg-Calve-Perthes disease of the hip is a condition of unknown etiology, but is considered to be an idiopathic avascular necrosis of the femoral head. It usually occurs around the ages of 3-10, more commonly in *males*. This source of hip pain can confuse clinicians, who must differentiate it with septic arthritis of the hip. Symptoms can range from a painless limp to intermittent knee, hip, groin, or thigh pain. On exam one may note hip stiffness with a loss of internal rotation and abduction. On imaging (recommended AP pelvis and frog leg laterals) may depict medial joint space widening. A *"crescent sign"* may be noticed indicating secondary subchondral collapse. Secondary osteoarthritis is a common sequela. The main goal of treatment is to keep the femoral head contained, which can be done with a combination of activity restriction, partial weight bearing, and physical therapy. For older children or those not responding to non-operative treatment may utilize surgical intervention with femoral and/or pelvic osteotomy.

Slipped capital femoral epiphysis (SCFE) is a resulting slippage of the femoral head on the femoral neck. It usually occurs during the adolescent growth spurt (~ 12 years of age), particularly in children who are *obese* or have *endocrine abnormalities.* Severe pain in the hip and/or knee is the main presenting complaint. It is an important diagnosis to make due to the high association with *avascular necrosis* of the femoral head, especially those cases that are acute and unstable (*medial femoral circumflex artery* is susceptible). Clinically, when the patient has their legs dangling off of the

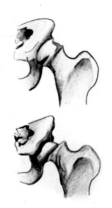

Figure 23: SCFE, stable (above), and unstable (below)

table, the sole of the affected foot faces the opposite foot. A physical exam maneuver may be the best diagnostic sign; with the patient supine, *flexing the thigh results in the femur rolling into external rotation and abduction.* Radiographic evaluation with *frog-leg* radiograph must be performed if the disorder is indicated. Assessing *Klein's line* can help determine whether there is a slip; A straight line drawn up the lateral surface of the femoral neck that does not touch the femoral head should suggest this

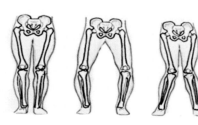

Figure 24: Normal (left), Genu varum (middle), genu valgum (right)

diagnosis. Treatment is generally operative, with *in situ* pinning of the physis with a screw, which arrests the progression of the slip (NO forceful reduction).

Varus and **valgus** deformities of the legs are commonly seen in children, and as a matter of fact may be normal to some extent (Figure 24). For example, genu (knee) varum is normal up to the age of 3. Varus refers to a displacement of the distal part of the extremity toward the midline. Valgus is defined as the opposite, with displacement of a distal part of the extremity away from the middle. An example is "knocked knees", in which the legs are valgus, pointing away from midline. Bow-legs would be knees that are in varus. Persistence of genu varum angular deformity into infant and adolescent stages is commonly termed **Blount's disease**, which is known to be secondary to a disturbed endochondral ossification of the medial proximal tibial growth plate. **Note:** genu varum may also occur secondary to rickets (seen as a widening of the physis on X-ray). Valgus deformities are seldom pathologic unless severe. Genu valgus is considered to be a normal variant between the ages of 4 and 8, when no treatment is needed. As bracing is usually not so effective, operative treatment with osteotomy and realignment can be done for both infants and adolescents. This essentially consists of fusing the lateral part of the physis to allow the medial half to "catch up."

Clubfoot (talipes equinovarus) is a deformity that is seen at birth, and has an association with early amniocentesis. This presents with both feet turned inward, plantar flexion of the ankle, adduction of the forefoot, and internal rotation of the tibia (Figure 25). As the name implies, this may represent the hoof of a horse. If left untreated, the patient may be forced to walk on the dorsolateral surface of the foot. Conservative treatment is generally successful,

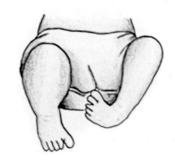

Figure 25: Talipes equinovarus

and involves using *serial plaster casts* that are changed every few weeks. Those who fail the cast

86

treatment may require surgery, typically between the ages of 9 and 12 months.

A commonly used mnemonic to remember the muscle contractures that lead to the characteristic deformity is **C.A.V.E.** This represents **C**avus of the midfoot, **A**dductus of the forefoot, **V**arus of the hindfoot, and **E**quinus of the hindfoot.

As parents always fear their loved ones will grow up to be crippled, a common complaint seen in an orthopedic clinic is **intoeing and outtoeing.** This is seldom pathologic, and usually spontaneously corrects itself. This may be due to a torsion of the femur or tibia. In femoral anteversion (most common cause of intoeing), a physical exam will show that on maximal internal rotation of the feet with the patient in the supine position, the knees point medially as to face each other. Treatment is *REASSURANCE.* Although that may be hard to accept for a worried parent, they can be comforted in knowing that if the child does not grow out of the deformity, surgical correction is still an option for the future.

If you were an athlete, you may have experienced **Osgood-Schlatter (apophysitis of the tibial tubercle)** first hand. Seen in teenagers, this presents with persistent pain/tenderness right over the tibial tubercle (Figure 26), and is aggravated by contraction of the quadriceps. Knee swelling is absent. Standard of therapy is RICE: Rest, Ice, Compress, Elevate. If conservative measures are unsuccessful, then patients may be treated with an extension or cylinder cast for 4 to 6 weeks, but this is generally not required.

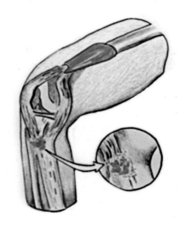

Figure 26: Osgood-Schlatter

Trauma

As an orthopedic surgeon, you will manage various sorts of trauma to the musculoskeletal system. Numerous trauma-scoring systems are utilized to allow for appropriate triage and classification of patients. These scoring systems help predict the outcomes of patients, allow for quality assurance, and also determine reimbursement in many cases. An important classification system based on anatomic criteria is called the **injury severity scale (ISS)**. This breaks down the body into 9 separate anatomic regions, each receiving a grade from 0 to 9 reflecting the caliber of the injury. The *three* most severely injured variables are used to calculate a final score by *adding up the sum of the squares*. For example, ISS = $A^2 + B^2 + C^2$, where A, B, and C are the most severely injured regions. The final score ranges from 1 to 75, with the stipulation that any single score of 6 warrants an automatic score of 75. A total score greater than 15 is associated with an approximate 10% mortality.

SIRS (systemic inflammatory response syndrome) is a nonspecific inflammatory condition that can occur secondary to various causes, the most common being sepsis, but also from major accidental trauma. Clinically one may notice lability in the patient's vital signs and resultant organ dysfunction and failure, all secondary to the actions of an uncontrolled release of cytokines. To meet SIRS criteria, the patient must have 2 of the following:
- Fever > 100.4 or < 96.8
- Heart rate > 90
- Respiratory rate > 20
- White blood cell count >12,000 or <4,000

Fat embolism, a consequence of long bone fractures, primarily produces pulmonary and cerebral inflammation. This is important to keep in mind after trauma to long bones such as femur fractures. Fat embolism is characterized by hypoxia and confusion with an onset of 24-72 hours after long bone fractures (most commonly a femoral shaft fracture). Petechia and thrombocytopenia may also be noted (may present as skin lesions). Treatment consists of pulmonary support with oxygen and mechanical ventilation if necessary.

Compartment syndrome occurs in anatomical areas where muscle and tissue is bound by fascia and resultant swelling raises the pressure in the compartment to a point that blood flow is impeded. When the interstitial pressure exceeds capillary perfusion, muscle and nerve necrosis can eventually occur. This generally occurs when the compartment pressures *exceed 30 mmHg*, or if the pressure is within 30 mm Hg of the diastolic pressure. Although this can be measured by certain instruments (you will hear "Stryker needle" being used), compartment syndrome is a clinical diagnosis. The most commonly affected compartments are of the *legs* and the *forearms*, but can essentially occur anywhere (traumatic brain injury with an increase in intracranial pressure is technically considered a "compartment syndrome"). A history of trauma followed by increased rather than improving pain on muscle stretch is characteristic. Pain with passive stretch, pallor, pulselessness, paralysis, and paresthesias are the **5 P's** to remember. This is treated with urgent fasciotomy, which allows for swelling. Volkmann's contracture may be the end result if left untreated (Figure 18).

One of the more devastating results of trauma is an injury to the **spinal cord injury.** Usually irreversible, the mainstay of care is prevention. This is why we assume that all trauma victims have an unstable spine susceptible to cord injury, and keep the patients in a cervical collar, on a firm surface, and logroll them as necessary. **Note:** X-ray and CT scan may not show ligamentous instability. In an awake and alert patient *with* pain or midline tenderness plus normal x-ray findings, lateral films in flexion and extension can be used to evaluate for subluxation of the vertebrae.

Depending on the mechanism of injury, it is important to assess for **nerve injuries.** Such damage can be characterized by various terms, including *neuropraxia, axonotmesis,* and *neuronotmesis:*

Neuropraxia – bruising of the nerve, recovers in minutes to days (similar to a concussion of the brain)
Axonotmesis – significant bruise where axons break down, but can grow back because Schwann cells and the endoneurium are left intact. Grows back at ~ 1 mm/day.
Neuronotmesis – complete transection of the nerve.

It is important to assess for sensory, motor, and reflex function of the suspected injured nerve. Pinprick is supposed to be a more sensitive test than light touch. It is also of benefit to repair associated tendon lacerations corresponding to the nerve. In regard to treatment, a transection repair can be done to convert it from a neuronotmesis to an axonotmesis with potential for recovery. If important enough, sacrificing a less important nerve may be carried out to graft a significantly injured nerve.

Pelvic Fractures are potentially life-threatening and should be suspected in high-energy trauma, as from falls or MVCs; they have a high association with injuries to other organ systems. Thus, as with all trauma cases, primary assessment of immediate life-threatening injuries (ABC's) should be initiated. Considering the Young & Burgess classification below, AP compression fractures are often associated with abdominal injury. LC compression fractures are often associated with brain injury. Pelvic fractures may also be associated with retroperitoneal hemorrhage, resulting in *massive intravascular volume loss.* It is understood that up to 6 units of blood can accumulate in the pelvis! This is commonly secondary to injury of the venous plexus in the posterior pelvis or due to large vessel injuries. Assessment for neurologic injury is also essential as the lumbosacral plexus and nerve roots are susceptible structures, especially with penetrating trauma. Additionally, there may be corresponding bladder, urethral, and bowel injuries in such cases, and so require a multidisciplinary approach. **Note**: these may not be so apparent in an unconscious patient and so a high index of suspicion is required.

> **Trendelenburg sign** – Have patient stand and lift one leg; on the flexed side, the pelvis should elevate. Failure or if pelvis falls indicates abductor or gluteus medius (superior gluteal nerve) dysfunction on planted side

Pelvic fractures are notoriously difficult to treat and require an algorithmic approach. *External fixation* as with a pelvic binder can be very helpful in decreasing additional injury and inducing/maintaining tamponade. **Note:** Exceptions to the association with high-energy trauma are non-threatening fractures of the pubic rami resulting from low energy falls in osteoporotic patients (treated non-operatively). Understanding the injuries involving the pelvis is a rather complex topic and may require extra time and sources.

In regards to radiographic evaluation, there are a few specific views to take note of:

- Pelvic **inlet** view is taken AP with the beam 45 degrees caudad. This will help show *posterior displacement* or *pubic symphysis widening* with pelvic ring fractures.
- Pelvic **outlet** view is taken AP with the beam 45 degrees cephalad. This also shows pelvic ring fractures, but may delineate a *superior displacement*.
- **Judet** views are used to characterize *acetabular fractures*. This is taken with the beam obliquely facing the affected hip, at a level of about 45 degrees. There are two kinds, "iliac oblique" and "obturator oblique." Iliac oblique is taken by placing a bump under the contralateral hip, and an obturator oblique is taken with a bump under the ipsilateral hip. Note: instead of a bump, the beam can be moved instead. What these specific judet views depict can be remembered by the mnemonic "PIC & POW"; The "I" and "O" stand for iliac and obturator respectively, and the "C" and "W" stand for column and wall, respectively.
- There are 6 cardinal lines to identify on a pelvic radiograph. If any of these seem disrupted or out of the ordinary, then further investigation may be required. The 6 lines are as follow:
  - o Ilioischial line
  - o Iliopectineal line
  - o "Tear drop"
  - o Roof of the acetabulum
  - o Anterior wall of the acetabulum
  - o Posterior wall of the acetabulum

The Young and Burgess classification system is the one that is commonly used for pelvic fractures and organizes such lesions based on the mechanism of injury

- APC (anterior-posterior compression)
  - I – pubic symphysis diastasis < 2.5 cm
  - II – pubic symphisis diastasis > 2.5 cm PLUS anterior SI joint disruption
  - III – complete separation of anterior and posterior pelvis, allowing for significant rotational instability
- LC (Lateral compression)
  - I – Compression of SI joint PLUS ipsilateral pubic ramus fracture
  - II – iliac wing fracture
  - III – contralateral APC 3 ("windswept pelvis")

When assessing an AP pelvis, it may help to start at the top and use a systematic approach. You will learn which method works best for you, but in order to make sure you do not miss any potentially significant pathology it is important to work systematically as with anything. Here is an example: First, look at L5. Look out for any disruption/avulsion of the transverse processes... this indicates disruption of the posterior ligaments. This is important because the posterior ligaments are some of the strongest in the pelvis and if they are disrupted, then you are working with a high-energy injury. Then proceed to look at the SI joint. If the superior aspect has disruption, this indicates posterior involvement (automatic APC-3 classification). Inferior widening of the SI joint indicates anterior disruption. Then assess the pubic symphisis for any diastasis. If there is widening there, then it is classified as an automatic APC. If there is only a fracture of the ramus, it is characterized as LC-1. Crest fractures are considered LC-2.

As I mentioned before, injuries to the pelvis are significant, but they are also complex. If you are going to be spending time at a trauma center then understanding and learning pelvic anatomy and pathology is very important. Also important to understand would be tibial plateau and shaft fractures as these commonly occur secondary to trauma. Another caveat: In trauma cases, fracture fragments pose an issue to the treating physician. These fragments are often devascularized and may become infected if the fracture was open or was treated surgically. The sequestered bone usually needs to be removed, and is often difficult to locate and resect.

Joint Replacement

An advancement in medicine that has significantly decreased disability in the world is the advent of joint replacements, particularly those of the knees and hips. This can be termed a total (hip) arthroplasty or a hemiarthroplasty depending on the procedure. The procedure used is determined by certain indications. A *hemiarthroplasty* is when a part of the joint is replaced, whereas a *total* consists of replacing the entire joint. For example, a hemiarthroplasty of the hip is replacing just the femoral head whereas a total replaces the hip AND the acetabulum. Joints are relatively complex structures, and the details of the procedure are even more intricate. From a beginner's level it is most important to understand the indications and contraindications to joint replacements, as well as familiarize yourself with the various surgical approaches (for all surgeries, really) and any anatomical considerations, as you may be scrubbing into several of these cases.

Tumors

In brief, most bone tumors are non-malignant, although there are cancerous types that are rapidly life-threatening. Although musculoskeletal oncology is an elaborate subject in itself, there are a few basic facts that are important to understand. First off, primary bone tumors are usually rare after the 3rd decade, in which case metastasis is probable. Musculoskeletal tumors generally present as pain and swelling without any significant trauma to the area. They may also cause fractures from unusual mechanisms of injury that would not normally cause a fracture. The malignant types of soft tissue tumors are most often beneath the fascia, and may be accompanied by constitutional symptoms such as malaise, anorexia, weight loss etc. The most

Mnemonic: **Pb KTL** (lead kettle) – common origins of bony mets

common bone lesions are bony metastasis, usually from a primary prostate, breast, kidney, thyroid, or lung source (mnemonic: Pb KTL). **Note:** tumors of the bone from metastasis may be described by the patient as being *worse at night.* The most vascular marrow is in the central part of the body, and so metastases often occur in the axial skeleton, the hips, and the shoulders. *Uniquely, prostate metastases cause BLASTIC lesions, which appear dense on x-ray, compared to the more common lytic lesion.*

The most common primary malignant bone tumor is **osteogenic sarcoma (osteosarcoma).** It arises in rapidly growing bone, near the rapidly growing physes in adolescents. Interestingly, constitutional symptoms such as fever, malaise, and weight loss are often absent. Regarding laboratory work, LDH and alkaline phosphatase will be elevated from the turnover of damaged osteocytes. Predisposing factors include Paget's disease of bone (older patients), radiation, and familial retinoblastoma. Lesions are commonly found in the metaphyses of long bones, around the distal femur/proximal tibia region. On x-ray this presents with a classic "sunburst pattern" or a "codman's triangle" from the reactive elevation of the periosteum. This tumor is considered aggressive, and is treated with surgical en bloc resection with limb salvage (often with difficult reconstructions) and adjuvant chemotherapy.

The second most common primary malignant bone tumor is a

Ewing Sarcoma. It generally affects children around 5-15 years of age, and grows in the *diaphysis* of long bones. The classic pattern seen on x-rays is the *"onion skinning"* type of periosteal reaction.

A common malignancy involving bone is **multiple myeloma.** Although this is a condition where plasma cell reproduction is unregulated, the bone marrow is particularly affected, as is the rest of the skeleton. This is a disease that occurs in older adults, more commonly in African Americans and males. Myeloma cells come from uncontrollable plasma cells, which tend to involve the entire skeleton, and infiltrate virtually all of a patient's bone marrow. *X-ray* images show "lytic lesions" (in contrast to blastic lesions as seen in prostate cancer), which look like holes that have been "punched out." Bone scan may not be a good way to locate these lesions as they do not have sclerotic, reactive borders which are normally seen in destructive lesions. Patients complain of bone pain and other constitutional symptoms. On laboratory findings, patients may have hyper**C**alcemia, **R**enal failure, **A**nemia (normocytic, normochromic)/pancytopenia, and **B**one lesions **(Mnemonic: C.R.A.B).** This cancer is also associated with an increased susceptibility to infection (abnormal immunoglobulins), and amyloidosis. Currently not curable, the treatment consists of a combination of chemotherapy with Melphalan and Prednisone, radiation therapy, and supportive care. If chemotherapy fails, Thalidomide may be used. If the patient is younger than 70 years of age and a fair candidate, stem cell transplant is an excellent option. The use of surgery is generally used to decrease pain and to maintain function rather than to cure the disease.

As malignant lesions can make the surrounding bone more susceptible to fractures, it is important to consider when prophylactic nailing can be of benefit. This is standardly assessed using the **Mirel's criteria.** This is based off of 4 factors: *size, lesion type, location,* and *pain.* Each of these are graded from 1-3, and depending on what the factors add up to, *if the sum is >8, then prophylactic fixation* may be indicated.

Mirel's criteria			
Score	**1**	**2**	**3**
Site	Upper limb	Lower limb	peritrochanteric
Pain	Mild	Moderate	Severe
Lesion type	Blastic	Mixed	Lytic
Size	< 1/3 canal	1/3 - 2/3	> 2/3

Practice Questions

1.   Interpret this x-ray:

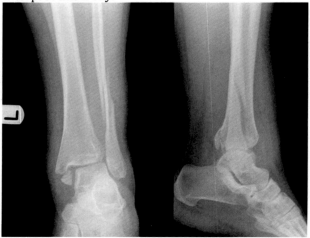

2.   A 43-year-old male presents with a severely comminuted open fracture of the proximal 1/3 of the tibia secondary to a gunshot wound. What antibiotic should you prophylactically treat with (a)? What if the wound is clearly not sterile, which antibiotic would you add(b)? What if you are still not satisfied with coverage and suspect significant contamination(c)?

3.   As you are examining a 24-year-old female with a new ulnar shaft fracture after a fall, she complains that the extremity is becoming progressively more painful and more tense, and "it seems to be getting paler." The patient complains of pain on passive extension of the fingers and wrist, and the pulses are normal. What is the diagnosis?

4.   What should you particularly look for to assess muscle viability when you perform a fasciotomy?

5.   Name 3 reasons fractures should be reduced.

6. When reducing a dislocation, what are the 3 basic steps to keep in mind regardless of involved joint?

7. What type of bone is most affected in osteoporosis?

8. A 17-year-old male was playing basketball when he jumped up for a rebound and landed on his opponent's foot, rolling his ankle. On exam there is significant swelling and tenderness at the lateral aspect of the midfoot. The foot is able to be inverted beyond the anatomical barrier with a soft end-point. What is the grade of this sprain? Which ligament is definitely involved? What is the progression of ligaments injured after this one?

9. A 30-year-old male was riding his bike when he suddenly hit a pothole and came to a complete stop, and was thrown over the handlebars and landed on right shoulder with no support of his hands. On exam, you notice a step-off deformity on the right shoulder, but original plain film is normal. Suspecting an acromioclavicular dislocation, how can you better visualize whether there is an injury to the ligament? You diagnose a Grade 3 separation, how will you manage it?

10. 18-year-old boy presents to the ED after being unexpectedly tackled, complaining of left shoulder pain. The patient is holding their arm slightly abducted, and externally rotated. You notice a sensory deficit on the lateral aspect of the deltoid. Which nerve is potentially injured? How do you test its sensory function?

11. Patient comes in with a suspected posterior left shoulder dislocation. Which radiographic view is key to diagnosis, and what is the technique for how it is taken?

12. Patient mentions this is his 3rd shoulder dislocation. You are suspecting a humeral avulsion of the glenohumeral ligament from the recurrent dislocations. Which ligament is most likely to be affected?

13. In the setting of a shoulder dislocation, what is the term given to the avulsion of the anteroinferior glenoid rim? What is the associated lesion on the humerus and where does it occur?

14. You are suspecting a rotator cuff tear in a patient who is unable to lift the dorsum of their hand off of the small of their back. What is this provocative test and which muscle is it testing?

15. Weakness of which muscle causes *lateral* winging of the scapula, and which nerve is involved?

16. In humeral shaft fractures, which nerve is particularly susceptible to injury due to its location?

17. Proximal humerus fractures put which nerve at risk for injury?

18. Which ligament fails first in a posterior elbow dislocation? What is the "terrible triad" associated with this injury?

19. The anterior bundle of the medial collateral ligament is the most important structure in preventing excess valgus stress of the elbow. Where does this structure attach?

20. Inflammation of which tendon is known to cause lateral epicondylitis? What is the origin of this muscle?

21. A fracture of the proximal ulna with an associated radial head dislocation is called _____. The classification system used for such injuries is _____

22. Name the distal radius fracture with dorsal displacement (volar angulation)

23. Name the distal radius fracture with volar angulation

24. Name the distal radius fracture associated with disruption of the radiocarpal joint (fracture-dislocation), deeming it intra-articular in nature.

25. What are the normal tolerances for the following values when assessing a Colles' fracture...Radial inclination? Radial height? Volar tilt?

26. How do you measure carpal alignment after reducing a distal radius fracture?

27. A 5-year-old male presents with a fall on an outstretched hand with pain at the elbow. Radiograph demonstrates a radial head fracture. The stability of what structure is essential in evaluation of this patient's extremity?

28. Name the contents of the carpal tunnel.

29. Patient presents with wrist pain. There is tenderness at the anatomical snuffbox. AP and lateral radiographs are negative. What is the suspected fracture, what is the technique for the view to better assess the injury?

30. What is the blood supply to the scaphoid bone, and what is its significance?

31. What is the Terry Thomas sign when assessing a scapholunate dislocation?

32. What is the significance of interpreting Shenton's line when assessing a radiograph of the hip in a suspected hip dislocation?

33. Using the Thompson classification, what classification of injury is a posterior hip dislocation with a comminuted acetabular fracture?

34. As posterior hip dislocations are orthopedic emergencies, what is the upper ideal limit for which reduction should take place? Why?

35. What is the main supply of the femoral head? From which vessel does this originate?

36. What is the name of the avulsion fracture of the ankle that is caused by rupture by the AITFL from the tibia? What is its corresponding lesion on the fibula?

37. When assessing an ankle injury for syndesmotic injury, what are the radiographic measurements to take into consideration for the following: tibiofibular overlap? Medial clear space?

38. Name 3 options for treatment of a distal radius fracture.

39. Name the 4 Kanavel signs that are indicative of purulent flexor tenosynovitis

40. A Jones fracture of the 5th metatarsal base is defined by injury to which zone? What is its significance?

41. A zone 1 fracture of the 5th metatarsal is what type of fracture and is associated with which muscle?

42. When assessing a fracture of the proximal humerus, what constitutes a "part" according to the Neer classification? Are there any exceptions?

43. A Supination-external rotation mechanism fracture of the ankle is associated with what type and pattern of fracture at the distal fibula? This is associated with which Weber classification?

44. List the order of ossification for the parts of the elbow, with the corresponding ages.

45. What bundles make up the ACL? What is its blood supply?

46. What is the most sensitive test for carpal tunnel syndrome?

47. What is the most sensitive test for ACL rupture?

48. Name 3 factors that make an intertrochanteric fracture unstable.

49. When placing a sliding hip screw, what is tip-to-apex distance that indicates adequate placement? How is it measured?

50. What is the rotator interval? What does it consist of?

51. What is the first bone to ossify and last bone to fuse?

52. How are SLAP tears of the shoulder graded from 1-4? Which types can be repaired?

53. Where exactly do Achilles tendon ruptures occur? How do you manage these patients in the emergency room?

54. How do you test for the most commonly torn rotator cuff muscle?

55. How do you differentiate between a Garden 3 and a Garden 4 hip fracture on radiograph?

56. Define neuropraxia.

57. Which nerve is most commonly injured in a pediatric supracondylar fracture of the humerus?

58. What are the acceptable tolerances for humeral shaft fractures?

59. You are performing an ORIF of a lateral malleolus fracture. During your approach, which nerve should you be aware of, and at which particular location?

60. The Allman classification of clavicle fractures is based on 3 separate groups (1 = medial, 2 = distal, 3 = proximal). What are the subparts of the group 2 fractures?

61. What are the coracoclavicular ligaments, and which is stronger?

62. Which band of the AC ligament is strongest?

63. What are the indications for surgery in a clavicle fracture?

64. Name the eponym and the parts for the classification for supracondylar fractures of the humerus

65. Which Weber ankle fracture is associated with a vertical fracture of the medial malleolus?

66. Which type of tibial plateau fracture is associated with vascular injury?

67. If a patient present with excruciating heel pain suspecting a calcaneus fracture, what other part of the body should be assessed?

68. What radiographs are essential to a trauma workup?

69. What does a bucket handle meniscal tear represent radiographically?

70. What is the pathognomonic avulsion lesion associated with an ACL tear?

71. List the pattern of instability in perilunate dislocations.

72. What is the scapholunate distance that indicates instability?

73. What are the 3 areas of the femoral neck where fractures can occur? Is there one that is treated as it is an intertrochanteric fracture?

74. What is Wolff's law?

75. What is the eponym for a fracture of the distal 1/3 of the humerus? What neurovascular injury is commonly associated with it?

76. A 7-year-old boy presents with elbow pain. Radiograph shows a displaced posterior fat pad? What does this suggest?

77. What is an Essex-Lopresti injury of the arm?

78. 48-year-old male presents after motorcycle accident with an open fracture of the tibia. The laceration is about 4 cm in size. There is no vascular injury, but there is inadequate soft tissue coverage. What type of Gustilo-Anderson injury does this fall under?

79. According to the Rockwood grading for AC separations, what type of an injury includes both the AC and CC joints, with posterior displacement of the distal clavicle?

80. What are the deforming forces on the proximal fragment in a fracture to the femoral shaft?

81. Patient comes in with shoulder pain. You watch as the attending flexes the patient's shoulder to 90 degrees, adducts slightly about 10 degrees, and internally rotates the arm so the thumb is facing down. The patient is then asked to resist a downward force placed by the physician. What is this provocative test called and what is it assessing for?

82. What are 3 names that have been used to describe a fracture of the distal 1/3 of the radius with an associated disruption of the DRUJ?

83. In a clavicle fracture, what are the deforming forces on the medial fragment? Lateral fragment?

84. Name the 4 radiographic findings that indicate osteoarthritis.

85. During a medial approach to the ankle, specifically the posterior aspect of the medial malleolus, what neurovascular structures should be observed for?

86. Which nerve root is responsible for the Achilles reflex? What is its sensory innervation?

87. A new mother comes in with pain in her hand. Flexion of her thumb with ulnar deviation causes a pain at the radial side of the base of her thumb. What is the name of the provocative test, and what is her most likely diagnosis?

88. Which rotator cuff muscles are responsible for external rotation of the shoulder?

89. Which rotator cuff muscle attaches to the lesser tuberosity of the humerus?

90. A secretary for a busy law firm comes in with elbow pain. She mentions she is typing on her computer constantly, and denies having time to exercise in any way. With the elbow flexed, resistance to middle finger extension does no illicit pain. With the elbow fully extended, the same resistance to finger extension reproduces her pain. Which tendon is most likely involved in her condition?

91. A tourist comes to your office saying his job from his homeland consists of wringing birds necks. A tender prominence is noted around the medial base of the thumb. What is the name of this lesion? What causes this?

92. You are assessing a mechanical cause for your patient's hip dislocation and you decide to measure the "Q-angle." How is this measured?

93. What is a "snowboarders fracture"?

94. What is the most common offending organism in osteomyelitis?

95. Which radiographic line is helpful in diagnosing a SCFE (assessing whether it intersects the epiphysis)?

96. A 15-year-old boy comes in with his mother because of "bilateral knee pain." The patient mentions he is very active with seasonal sports, and he recently started playing competitive basketball. The patient states that the pain gets worse with exercises, particularly those involving flexion. On exam, there are two prominent, tender areas below the patella around the anterior tibial tubercle. Imaging is unremarkable. What is the most likely diagnosis?

97. What is the eponym for an avulsion fracture of the posterior malleolus?

98. List the 5 P's that suggest compartment syndrome.

99. A 79-year-old patient presents with a sudden onset of right hip pain after a fall. X-ray shows a periprosthetic fracture that is around the stem of the prosthetic implant. What is the name of the classification system used, and what type does this fall under?

Answers

1. *2 views, AP & Lateral of a left ankle, in a skeletally mature individual, demonstrating a spiral fracture of the distal fibula, with a transverse, displaced fracture of the medial malleolus, and evidence of syndesmotic disruption.

2.
   a. 1st generation cephalosporin (i.e. Cefazolin)
   b. Aminoglycoside
   c. Penicillin
      i. If allergic, give metronidazole

3. Compartment syndrome; remember the 5 P's – Pallor, pulselessness, paralysis, pain, paresthesias. Keep in mind that pulses may be the last factor to decrease

4. 4 C's – Color, consistency, capacity to bleed, contractility

5.
   a. Decrease soft tissue injury
   b. Patient comfort
   c. Reduce neurovascular injury

6. Accentuate the deformity, place traction, reverse the mechanism of injury

7. Cancellous bone

8.
   a. Grade 3
   b. Anterior talofibular ligament
   c. Calcaneofibular ligament → posterior talofibular

9.
   a. Stress view with weights in both hands
   b. Treat it with a sling, early range of motion, physical therapy

10.
   a. Axillary nerve
   b. Sensation to the lateral aspect of the shoulder

11. Axillary view – patient is supine, arm is abducted, and beam is aimed at the axilla.

12. Inferior glenohumeral ligament

13.
   a. Bankart lesion
   b. Hill Sachs lesion – occurs on the posterior aspect of the humeral head

14. Lift off test; Subscapularis muscle

15. Trapezius; Spinal accessory nerve

16. Radial nerve, as it crosses superficially through the spiral groove

17. Axillary nerve

18.
   a. Lateral collateral ligament;
   b. Radial head fracture, coronoid tip fracture, elbow dislocation

19. Sublime tubercle of the coranoid process

20. Extensor carpi radialis brevis; lateral epicondyle

21. Monteggia lesion; Bado classification

22. Colles' fracture

23. Smith's fracture

24. Barton's fracture

25.
- a. Radial inclination - 23 degrees
- b. Radial height - 11 mm
- c. Volar tilt - 11 degrees

26. Intersection on a lateral radiograph of the line through the radial shaft and one through the capitate. If it intersects within the carpus, then it is adequately aligned.

27. Distal radioulnar joint

28. *The median nerve, flexor digitorum profundus tendons, flexor digitorum superficialis tendons, and the flexor pollicis longus tendon.*

29. Scaphoid fracture; Wrist extension with ulnar deviation

30. Dorsal carpal branch of the radial artery; it is retrograde running distal to proximal, making it susceptible to avascular necrosis.

31. Widening of scapholunate space greater than 3 mm.

32. Possible associated femoral neck fracture

33. Thompson 3

34. 6 hours max; avascular necrosis of the femoral head

35. Medial femoral circumflex artery; profunda (deep) femoral artery

36.
- a. Tillaux fracture
- b. Lefort-Wagstaffe

37.
- a. Tib-fib overlap should be at least 10mm
- b. Medial clear space should be < 5mm

38.
- a. Non-operative with a splint/cast
- b. Percutaneous pinning

    c.   Volar plate and screws
    d.   External fixation

39.
    a.   Passive flexion
    b.   Pain with extension
    c.   Tenderness at the synovial sheath
    d.   Fusiform swelling

40. Zone 2; It is a watershed area, making it susceptible to nonunion

41. Avulsion fracture caused by the peroneus brevis muscle

42.
    a.   1 cm displacement or 45 degree angulation
    b.   The grater tuberosity is considered a part with as little as 5 mm displacement

43.
    a.   A spiral fracture of the distal fibula, running from anteroinferior to posterosuperior
    b.   Supination external rotation (by Lauge Hansen classification) corresponds to a Weber 2 lesion (involvement at the level of the plafond)

44. Capitellum (1-year-old) → radial head (3) → medial epicondyle (5) → trochlea (7) → Olecranon (9) → lateral epicondyle (11)

45.
    a.   Anteromedial and posterolateral bundles
    b.   Middle geniculate artery

46. Durkan's compression test

47. Lachman's test

48.
    a.   Reverse obliquity pattern
    b.   Subtrochanteric extension

    c. Calcar (posteromedial cortex) comminution

49.

    a. < 25 mm
    b. The sum of the measurements on both AP and lateral films of the hip of the distance between the tip of the screw to the apex of the femoral head.

50.

    a. The space between the tendons of the supraspinatus and subscapularis
    b. Consists of the coracohumeral ligament, superior glenohumeral ligament, and the long head of the biceps

51. Clavicle

52.

    a. 1 - Fraying
    b. 2 - Avulsion
    c. 3 - Bucket handle tear
    d. 4 - Bucket handle tear with associated bicep detachment
    e. Types 2 & 4 can be repaired
    f. Types 1 & 3 can be debrided

53.

    a. ~ 3cm above its insertion on the posterior tuberosity
    b. Cast them in equuinus

54. The supraspinatus is tested using the Jobe's empty can test. This is done by having the patient abduct the arm to 90 degrees and internally rotate the arm so the thumb is facing down. The patient is then asked to resist a downward force by the physician. Weakness in doing this indicates a possible weakness of the supraspinatus muscle.

55. Assess the trabecular lines. They are parallel in Garden 4, and perpendicular in Garden 3.

56. When bruising occurs to a nerve, to the minor extent of injury that recovery occurs in minutes to days

57. Anterior interosseus nerve (AIN)

58.
    a.   20 degrees of AP angulation
    b.   30 degrees of varus/valgus angulation
    c.   3 cm shortening

59. Superficial peroneal nerve; approximately 12 cm superior to the lateral malleolus

60.
    a.   Distal or interligamentous to the coracoclavicular ligaments
    b.   Proximal to the coracoclavicular ligaments
    c.   Involvement of the AC joint

61. Conoid (stronger) and trapezoid

62. Superior ligament

63.
    a.   Open fracture
    b.   Skin tenting (potential conversion to open)
    c.   Neurovascular compromise (brachial plexus)
    d.   Displacement/shortening of >2mm

64. Gartland classification
       i.   Nondisplaced
      ii.   Displaced with intact posterior cortex
     iii.   Displaced posterior cortex

65. Weber Type A

66. That involving the medial aspect (Schatzker Type 4)

67. Spine

68.

a. Chest x-ray
b. Pelvis x-ray
c. Lateral C-spine

69. "Double PCL sign"

70. Segond fracture (avulsion of the lateral tibia)

71.
a. Scapholunate dysjunction
b. Lunocapitate
c. Lunotriquetrum
d. Perilunate dislocation

72. >3mm

73. Basicervical, transcervical, subcapital... A basicervical fracture is treated as an intertrochanteric fracture

74. It is the theory that bone/trabeculae will adapt to the external forces that are placed on it

75.
a. Holstein-Lewis
b. Radial nerve palsy

76. Nondisplaced supracondylar fracture of the humerus

77. Radial head fracture + interosseus membrane disruption + DRUJ disruption

78. 3B

79. Type 4

80.
a. The gluteus medius and minimus place an abducting force
b. Iliopsoas flexes the segment

81.
a. O'brien's test

      b. SLAP tear (integrity of the superior labrum)

82.
      a. Galleazzi fracture
      b. Fracture of necessity
      c. Piedmont fracture

83.
      a. The sternocleidomastoid (SCM) and trapezius muscles displace the medial fragment posterosuperiorly, and the pectoralis major muscle pulls the lateral fragment inferomedially.

84.
      a. Osteophytes
      b. Subchondral cysts
      c. Joint space narrowing
      d. Sclerosis

85.
      a. Posterior tibial artery
      b. Tibial nerve

86.
      a. S1
      b. Lateral and plantar aspects of the foot

87.
      a. Finklestein test
      b. DeQuervian's tenosynovitis

88. Infraspinatus & Teres minor

89. Subscapularis

90. This is indicative of lateral epicondylitis. The tendon most likely to be involved is the ECRB

91.
      a. Stener lesion from "Gamekeeper's thumb"
      b. Retraction of the torn ulnar collateral ligament into the adductor pollicis

92. *Q-angle* is defined by a line drawn from the ASIS through the center of the patella, with a second line from the center

of the patella to the tibial tubercle. A normal Q angle is around 15 degrees (females may have a greater angle).

93. One of the lateral process of the talus

94. *Staph Aureus*

95. Klein's line

96. Osgood-Schlatter disease

97. Curbstone fracture

98.
   a. Pain out of proportion to physical findings/pain with passive stretch
   b. Pallor
   c. Paresthesias
   d. Paralysis
   e. Pulselessness

99. Vancouver classification – Type B

Quick Reference

Upper Extremity tests:
- PIN (Radial n.) – "Thumbs up"
- AIN (Median n.) – "Okay sign"
- Ulnar n. – spread fingers out

Also remember the common sensory and motor innervations of the extremities:
- Axillary n.
  - Motor = Deltoid & Teres minor
  - Sensory = Lateral upper arm
- Musculocutaneous n.
  - Motor = Biceps, brachialis, coracobrachialis
  - Sensory = Lateral forearm
- Tibial n.
  - Motor = Plantar flexion, knee flexion, toe flexion
  - Sensory = foot Sole
- Superficial peroneal n.
  - Motor = Ankle EVERSION
  - Sensory = foot Dorsum
- Deep peroneal n.
  - Motor: Dorsiflexion & inversion & toe extension
  - Sensory = 1st toe web space

Made in the USA
San Bernardino, CA
23 March 2019